Diet or ... ek. The weight-l... iving plan that anyone can follow.

This small book provides a practical guide to following the 5:2 diet. Written in an easy-to-follow and friendly style by Jacqueline Whitehart. Jacqueline was one of the first followers of what is now known as the 5:2 diet. She continues to follow the diet and is one of its most well-regarded advocates.

This practical book gives you all the advice and tips you need to get started on this diet. There's week-by-week updates on what and when you should eat. Plus tips and motivation right when you need it.

Jacqueline has devised a full range of over 100 fantastic, filling recipes. From breakfasts to snacks, light lunches and dinners. The recipes are expertly balanced with plenty of protein and moderate complex carbohydrates. They're all designed to fill you up and stave off hunger pangs.

The 5:2 diet has a simple basis. 2 days per week you eat a quarter of your normal recommended calories – that's 500 for women and 650 for men. These are your fasting days. The other 5 days are feast days, when you can eat what you like. Sounds easy? That's because it is.

Read on to get started on a healthier, lighter future.

Important note
The information and advice contained in this book are intended as a general guide to dieting and healthy eating and are not specific to individuals or their particular circumstances. This book is not intended to replace treatment by a qualified practitioner. Neither the authors nor the publishers can be held responsible for claims arising from inappropriate use of any dietary regime. Do not attempt self-diagnosis or self-treatment for serious or long-term conditions without consulting a medical professional or qualified practitioner.

First published in Great Britain in 2012 by

Pepik Ltd

enquiries@pepik.com

www.pepik.com

Contents

Introduction

For two non-consecutive days each week you follow a restricted calorie diet – that's 500 calories for women and 650 for men. The other five days a week you eat whatever you like.

As well as being an excellent way to lose weight the long-term health benefits of this diet are impressive. Following the 5:2 diet can reduce cholesterol levels, cut your risk of diabetes, lower your cancer risk and delay the onset of Alzheimer's. Find out the latest research results in the "How the 5:2 diet can help you live longer" chapter of this book.

I may be an expert dieter but I am definitely not a scientist so I have chosen to concentrate on the weight-loss element of the diet. You shouldn't forget that by following the 5:2 diet you may well be extending your good health for longer into old age.

As with all diets you should seek advice from a health professional before starting. This is especially true if you have any particular health concerns. This diet is definitely **not** recommended if you are pregnant or breast-feeding, diabetic or hyperglycaemic.

As a typical working mum I've always found a lack of time and motivation for diets. They just simply don't fit in with a busy lifestyle, my love of salt and vinegar crisps and the desire for a glass of wine after a hard day wrangling kids. So I've tried many things: the Atkins diet, calorie counting, gym membership.. to name only three. They all start off well and then slowly fade away as other things in life take priority.

But the 5:2 diet has been different. I came across the diet quite by chance and was so impressed by the claimed health benefits that I decided it was worth a try. The weight-loss element of the diet was just one of the aspects that appealed.

Straight away I saw the benefits. Immediate weight-loss and increased energy. After only a week the fasting days became simple and easy to slot into my lifestyle. Now they hold no fear and I even find myself looking forward to them. I love the fact that for most of the week I can eat what I like and not worry about it.

Quite simply this diet has changed my life so much and given me so many benefits that I have, for the first time in my life, felt the need to share this breakthrough diet with as many people as possible. I hope it works as well for you as it has for me.

If **you** find success with this diet please consider leaving your story as a review on amazon.co.uk. This may help other people benefit from the 5:2 diet.

Yours,

Jacqueline

Jacqueline Whitehart, October 2012

Why the 5:2 diet?

The 5:2 diet is for you, for me, for everyone. It's proven to be easier to stick to than other diets. Why? Because its rules are so simple AND because you only diet two days a week. For five full days you are not on a diet. Because you know that following each day on which you diet you can eat normally the motivation to complete the diet day without giving in to temptation is high. And when you see yourself losing weight and still continuing to eat as normal 5 days a week it's easy to find the strength to carry on.

With the 5:2 diet you really can "**eat cake and lose weight too**".

There are three main benefits of the 5:2 diet. The first is of course losing weight, which is done gradually and safely, meaning the pounds stay off for good.

The second is that it is easy to follow and stick to; in fact, early stages of research into comparisons between this diet and others show that after a six week period a significantly higher proportion of 5:2 dieters were sticking to the diet than any other weight-loss plan. It is the knowledge that you only ever have to wait until the next morning that makes it so easy to keep going. It certainly works for me: I always look forward to my breakfast on the evening of my diet day, imagining the delights I can eat. But the strange thing is, when I wake up the next morning I'm not even particularly hungry.

The third is the most amazing health benefits that this simple diet seems to offer. It seems that the 5:2 diet can reduce the risks of some of the diseases we associate with ageing; in particular heart disease, some cancers and Alzheimer's. Because the effects of intermittent fasting, of which the 5:2 diet is one variant, have not been fully researched long-term we can't state or prove all of these benefits, but all the research done so far on the 5:2 (and other very similar diets such as Intermittent Fasting (IF), Alternate Day Fasting (ADF) and the Two-day diet) show promising results. Take a look at the chapter "How the 5:2 diet can help you live longer" if you want to find out about the existing research in more detail.

The 5:2 diet and me

Before I started the 5:2 diet I weighed in at just under 11 stone, size 14, with a BMI of 23.4. Not in the overweight category, but slowly and inexorably creeping towards it. Before I had children I was always around 10 stone but by the time I'd had my third child I found it close to impossible to shift the excess weight.

Four months after starting the 5:2 diet I was 10 stone 2 pounds. I am now a much happier size 12 with a BMI of 21.6.

Since then I've maintained my weight at approximately that level through fasting one or two days a week. I continue to eat healthily but without dieting on the other days.

Before I started this diet I thought I suffered with low blood sugar; I could never skip a meal and by lunchtime I would always be starving and grumpy. Within a couple of weeks of following the 5:2 diet I had noticed a huge difference. I follow Plan 1 for women, allowing myself a small snack for lunch and more often than not a stew and some green vegetables for my dinner (as this is something my whole family can enjoy). I've included all my favourites in the recipe section.

Getting started

There's no time like the present to get started with the 5:2 diet. If you are healthy and do not have any medical conditions such as diabetes then you are ready to go.

The principle rules of 5:2 dieting are simple. Twice a week you follow a calorie-restricted diet (500 calories for women and 650 for men) while the rest of the week you can eat whatever you like.

On your diet days you are shocking your body into breaking down more fat. On your non-diet days you eat what you like but it is virtually impossible to make up the missing calories. Research has shown that an average person eats at most 10-15% more than normal on the day following a diet day.

What's more it's incredibly simple to do. Once you get over some hunger pangs in the first week or two your body adapts to the restricted calories on your diet days, meaning the 5:2 diet is extremely easy to stick to in the long-term.

In this book I'll guide and encourage you through every step of the first few weeks. With menu plans and scrumptious recipe ideas you'll find the 5:2 diet easy to follow and stick with. So let's get started and plan your first day.

Choosing your diet days

At the start of each week you should see what days would fit in best with your schedule. Remember the days need to be non-consecutive. Obviously days where you have social arrangements, a meal out or drinks with friends planned should not be diet days. You should see this as one of the great advantages of this plan. You can still enjoy going out to restaurants, eating puddings guilt-free and generally enjoying life as it should be enjoyed.

For your fasting days you should choose the least social days on your calendar. They are likely to be work days – work is a great distraction from food – and days when you have plenty going on.

The only restriction on your diet days is that you must have a rest day between fasts. The diet days can change each week – making it the ultimate flexible diet. You just need to tick off two days each week as diet days and you will be right on track to some impressive health and weight-loss benefits.

In the first two weeks of the diet your diet days should also be relatively quiet days. Days when you don't have important meetings, are not doing anything too physical and when you are not likely to be exposed to a lot of nice food and cooking. This is because in the first 2 weeks of the diet you may suffer from hunger pangs, feel slightly light-headed at times and generally be in need of a spot of will-power. But rest assured, as each fasting day is completed successfully the next will be significantly easier. By week three diet days should become an easy and regular part of your routine, not holding you back at all.

When to eat, What to eat

Before you start on your first diet day it is wise to think about how best to manage your food over the day. To do this you need to think about your lifestyle and your body's needs. Here are a few questions that might help you decide what and when to eat.

- Are you working in an office?
- Are you busy during the day with little time to think about food?
- Are you time pressed so cooking is difficult?
- Are you exposed to unhealthy food during the day?
- Are you cranky if you miss breakfast?
- Do you feel most hungry in the evenings?
- When do you tend to get food cravings?

There are various ways in which to split your calories throughout the day; each one will be described in detail shortly. But as a general guide if you tend to be super busy during the day with no time to stop you should go for a breakfast and dinner option. But if you're in a rush in the morning and aren't particularly hungry first thing you should try an option with more food at lunch and dinner-time.

Menu planning

Here we must split into different plans for men and women. As men are allowed 650 calories on their diet days (compared to 500 calories for women) they have more options for what and when to eat. Rest assured ladies that they are not going to feel any less hungry than you.

Menu plans for women

Plan 1 (no breakfast)

Breakfast: Milky drink (2 cups tea or coffee with skimmed milk OR 100ml glass of skimmed or soya milk)

–

Lunch: light lunch or snack, totalling 150 calories

–

Dinner: main meal, totalling 300 calories

Plan 2 (no lunch)

Breakfast: up to 200 calories, including drinks

–

Lunch: NO LUNCH

–

Dinner: main meal, totalling 300 calories

Plan 3 (3 small meals)

Breakfast: up to 150 calories, including drinks

–

Lunch: up to 150 calories

–

Dinner: up to 200 calories

Ladies, you should choose which of these plans works for you best, or make up your own! Try it out using the detailed menu plans on the following pages for each option. All of the recipes are designed to be healthy and filling, helping you to stave off those hunger pangs.

If this looks scary or difficult, it's not – I, Jacqueline Whitehart, hater of diets with a shortage of will-power, totally promise! Your body soon adapts to the lower amount of calories and you definitely won't starve. Above all, remember that your reward is to eat what you like tomorrow AND still watch the weight fall off.

Menu plans for men

Plan A (no breakfast)

Breakfast: Milky drink (2 cups tea or coffee with skimmed milk or 100ml glass of skimmed or soya milk).

–

Lunch: up to 300 calories

–

Dinner: main meal, totalling 300 calories

Plan B (no lunch)

Breakfast: full breakfast, totalling up to 300 calories

–

Lunch: tiny snack (50 calories)

–

Dinner: main meal, totalling 300 calories

Plan C (3 small meals)

Breakfast: up to 150 calories, including drinks

–

Lunch: 200 calories

–

Dinner: main meal, totalling 300 calories

Following the menu planners

These menu planners have been put together based on the recipes in this book. The recipes have all been designed to be healthy, to fill you up and to stave off hunger pangs. The recipes are high in protein and complex (low GI) carbohydrates, while being low in fat. Some are designed to be prepared quickly and easily for one, others are designed to be cooked in bigger portions and either shared with the family or frozen in individual portions (practically all of the recipes here are freezer-friendly) so you have a perfect ready-to-eat meal in minutes without resorting to a ready-meal.

Talking of ready-meals, at the time I write this there is a range of ready-meals at Marks and Spencer that fits very well into the 5:2 diet. The range is called "Simply Fuller Longer" and they have over 50 recipes, many of which are under 300 calories. So if you want to skip cooking altogether or just swap in one of their dinners when you really can't face cooking, you can and should. Just bear in mind that you need to make sure that you stick to the recommended number of calories for each meal.

For men, this means that you could have one of their wraps or salads for lunch, followed by a ready meal for dinner (as long as both are under 300 calories and you've just had tea or coffee for breakfast).

For women, you could have a ready-meal for dinner (under 300 calories) or swap your lunch and dinner around and have a wrap or salad for lunch followed by a light snack in the evening.

Please remember that while M&S is an ideal quick fix they are expensive and NOTHING beats home cooking for a nutritious filling meal. The recipes in this book are designed to give you a great balance of protein and carbohydrates.

Menu plan 1 (for women, no breakfast)

Breakfast is strictly limited to 2 cups of tea or coffee made with skimmed milk OR one latte coffee made with skimmed milk (see recipes) OR a 100ml glass of skimmed milk. Total calories should be less than fifty for breakfast.

Week 1

	Lunch	Dinner	Cals
Day 1	Smoked salmon and cream cheese on oatcakes, **page 58** *169 cals*	Chicken with orange and black olives, **page 98** *284 cals*	453
Day 2	Spicy butternut squash soup, **page 74** *169 cals*	Scallops with garlic tomatoes, **page 109** *258 cals*	427

Week 2

	Lunch	Dinner	Cals
Day 1	Savoy cabbage and bacon soup, **page 58** *156 cals*	Beef in mushrooms and wine, **page 123** *294 cals*	450
Day 2	Oriental prawn and mushroom salad, **page 49** *151 cals*	Sticky Thai chicken with 2 new potatoes and broccoli, **page 94** *305 cals*	456

Week 3

	Lunch	Dinner	Cals
Day 1	Pastrami on rye, **page 57** *137 cals*	Sweet potato chilli with 25g basmati rice, **page 86** *300 cals*	437
Day 2	Italian bread salad, **page 50** *170 cals*	Chunky cod with tomatoes and spinach, **page 107** *248 cals*	418

Menu plan 2 (for women, no lunch)

The total calories per day on this plan add up to approximately 450 calories. This is to allow for 2 cups of tea or coffee with milk OR a tiny snack (e.g. a piece of fruit) at lunch.

Week 1

	Breakfast	Dinner	Cals
Day 1	Healthy fry up with baked beans, **page 45** *194 cals*	Chunky cod with tomatoes and spinach, **page 107** *248 cals*	442
Day 2	Ham omelette, **page 60** *198 cals*	One pot Vegetable Tagine, **page 89** *247 cals*	445

Week 2

	Breakfast	Dinner	Cals
Day 1	Baked beans on toast, **page 44** *172 cals*	Quick fried beef with Salsa Verde, **page 119** served with 100g green beans (35 cals) *259 cals*	431
Day 2	Porridge pot, **page 43** and an apple (53 cals) *179 cals*	Chicken in tomato sauce, **page 96** served with 100g broccoli (33 cals) *288 cals*	467

Week 3

	Breakfast	Dinner	Cals
Day 1	Home-made Granola, **page 45** made with 100ml skimmed milk *199 cals*	Sweet and sour pork, **page 118** served with 50g curly kale (16 cals) *234 cals*	433
Day 2	Healthy fry up, **page 44** *178 cals*	Salmon and cod fishcakes, **page 108** *256 cals*	434

Menu plan 3 (for women, 3 small meals)

Week 1

	Breakfast	Lunch	Dinner	Cals
Day 1	Natural yoghurt with kiwi, **page 42** *91 cals*	Oriental prawn and mushroom salad, **page 49** *151 cals*	Ramen soup with udon noodles, **page 77** *215 cals*	457
Day 2	Egg white omelette, **page 42** *57 cals*	Lentil, lemon and thyme soup, **page 71** *121 cals*	Creamy chicken curry, **page 95** with 20g basmati rice (70 cals) *315 cals*	493

Week 2

	Breakfast	Lunch	Dinner	Cals
Day 1	Porridge pot, **page 43** and an apple (53 cals) *179 cals*	Chargrilled vegetable salad, **page 48** *127 cals*	Portobello mushrooms with spinach and tomato, **page 85** *195 cals*	501
Day 2	Blackberry fool, **page 41** *45 cals*	Pastrami on rye, **page 57** *137 cals*	Autumn lamb stew **page 116** with 2 new potatoes and 80g peas *320 cals*	502

Week 3

	Breakfast	Lunch	Dinner	Cals
Day 1	Hot chocolate, **page 43** *102 cals*	Oatcake with peanut butter and tomato, **page 56** *97 cals*	Quick fried beef with Salsa Verde, **page 119** served with 100g green beans (35 cals) *259 cals*	458
Day 2	Egg white omelette, **page 42** *57 cals*	Spicy butternut squash soup, **page 74** *169 cals*	Scallops with garlic tomatoes, **page 109** *258 cals*	484

Menu plan A (for men, no breakfast)

Breakfast is strictly limited to 2 cups of tea or coffee made with skimmed milk OR one latte coffee made with skimmed milk (see recipes) OR a 100ml glass of skimmed milk. Total calories should be less than fifty for breakfast.

Week 1

	Lunch	Dinner	Cals
Day 1	Hearty ham soup, **page 78** *224 cals*	Lemon sole with a herb crust, **page 104** with 4 new potatoes and 50g spinach *334 cals*	558
Day 2	Roast chicken and pesto flatbread, **page 63** *241 cals*	Chilli con carne, **page 121** with 40g basmati rice *365 cals*	606

Week 2

	Lunch	Dinner	Cals
Day 1	Refried beans and goat's cheese hot wrap, **page 64** *268 cals*	Beef in mushrooms and wine, **page 123** with 100g broccoli *327 cals*	595
Day 2	Ham omelette, **page 60** with half slice granary bread *298 cals*	Chunky cod with tomatoes and spinach, **page 107** with 2 new potatoes *318 cals*	616

Week 3

	Lunch	Dinner	Cals
Day 1	Ramen soup with udon noodles, **page 77** *215 cals*	Creamy chicken curry, **page 95** with 40g basmati rice *376 cals*	591
Day 2	Two BLT flatbreads, **page 59** *346 cals*	Steamed salmon with Chinese vegetables, **page 112** *296 cals*	642

Menu plan B (for men, no lunch)

Where half slice of bread is listed this could be a whole slice of "diet" bread or ½ thick slice of wholemeal or granary bread.

Week 1

	Breakfast	Dinner	Cals
Day 1	Healthy fry up with baked beans, **page 45** with ½ slice granary toast *294 cals*	Fresh pesto cod, **page 105** with 4 new potatoes and 50g spinach *336 cals*	630
Day 2	Scrambled eggs with peppers and tomatoes, **page 46** *249 cals*	Chilli con carne, **page 121** with 40g basmati rice *365 cals*	614

Week 2

	Breakfast	Dinner	Cals
Day 1	Double portion of porridge pot, **page 43** *252 cals*	Chicken with Orange and black olives, **page 98** with 2 new potatoes and 100g broccoli *387 cals*	639
Day 2	Ham omelette, **page 60** with ½ slice granary bread *298 cals*	Steamed salmon with Chinese vegetables, **page 112** *296 cals*	594

Week 3

	Breakfast	Dinner	Cals
Day 1	2 BLT flatbreads, **page 59** *346 cals*	One pot Thai curry, **page 88** *242 cals*	588
Day 2	Healthy fry up, **page 44** with ½ slice granary bread *278 cals*	Quick fried beef with Salsa Verde, **page 119** with 2 new potatoes and 100g green beans *327 cals*	605

19

Menu plan C (for men, 3 small meals)

Week 1

	Breakfast	Lunch	Dinner	Cals
Day 1	Natural yoghurt with kiwi, **page 42** *91 cals*	Warm leek and lentil salad with goat's cheese, **page 54** *298 cals*	Sweet and sour pork, **page 118** with 100g broccoli *251 cals*	640
Day 2	Baked beans on toast, **page 44** *172 cals*	Prawn in sweet chilli sauce wrap, **page 63** *239 cals*	Portobello mushrooms with spinach and tomato, **page 85** *195 cals*	606

Week 2

	Breakfast	Lunch	Dinner	Cals
Day 1	Healthy fry up, **page 44** *178 cals*	Chargrilled vegetable salad, **page 48** *127 cals*	Paprika pork casserole, **page 124** with 50g spinach *319 cals*	624
Day 2	Porridge pot, **page 43** *126 cals*	Rye bread with taramasalata, **page 59** *195 cals*	Chicken with brown mushrooms, **page 97** with 50g kale *300 cals*	621

Week 3

	Breakfast	Lunch	Dinner	Cals
Day 1	Scrambled eggs with peppers and tomatoes, **page 46** *249 cals*	Ham or bacon salad, **page 48** *98 cals*	Scallops with garlic tomatoes, **page 109** *258 cals*	605
Day 2	Hot chocolate, **page 43** *102 cals*	Refried beans and goat's cheese hot wrap, **page 64** *268 cals*	Quick fried beef with Salsa Verde, **page 119** with 100g green beans *259 cals*	629

Frequently Asked Questions

Q: Can I have caffeinated drinks?

A: Yes

Do you drink coffee or tea or colas regularly every day? You are definitely not alone. I do NOT advise you to give them up, even on your diet days. Why? Because caffeine withdrawal is likely to give you headaches and make your fasting days miserable and harder. So unless you have other reasons to give up caffeine just work out your normal consumption and make sure you count all the calories you have in your caffeinated drinks.

There are lots of ways to get your normal caffeine hit without adding any calories. Black tea and coffee and diet colas/energy drinks are the obvious choice. The calories in these drinks are insignificant.

But if your preferred drink is tea or coffee with milk then don't cut it out. Just make sure you count the calories in each cup. You should also consider shifting to skimmed milk which has 35 cals per 100ml as opposed to semi-skimmed which has 49 cals per 100ml.

Finally, I must admit that my breakfast choice from the above list is ALWAYS a skinny latte. I make my own and have perfected the recipe over the years. I have included it in the recipes section of the book. For reference a short skinny latte from Starbucks is 67 cals and a tall skinny latte is 102 cals. Other coffee outlets are similar.

Q: Should I exercise as normal?

A: Not on your diet days

When you start the 5:2 diet you may be wondering what to do about your normal exercise routine. In the first few weeks at least you should not try and exercise on your diet days. This is for two reasons. Firstly, you may feel physically weaker on your fasting days when you start this diet – this wears off soon. Secondly, exercising will simply make you more hungry – something you want to avoid at this stage.

You do however have 5 non-diet days for whatever exercise routine you normally do (or don't!) follow.

Q: What about alcoholic drinks?

A: Not on your diet days

Alcoholic drinks contain plenty of calories and will probably make you feel light-headed on your diet days so it's worth steering clear of alcoholic drinks on these days. Of course you're free to do what you want on the other 5 days.

Q: What should I eat on a feast (non-diet) day?

A: Whatever you like

The first rule for feast days is there are no rules! You can eat what you like and really enjoy it. This is your reward for the fast day before. Your body will regulate itself and even on the day after a fast day you'll at most eat 10% - 15% more than normal.

Be aware that on the first day after a fast day the breakfast that you've been looking forward to may be a bit of a let down. You'll be surprised that you cannot manage to eat as much as you thought you wanted. You may also feel rather tired and lethargic that first feast day. This is just your body compensating for the fast day. As your body gets used to fasting this won't happen and feast days will be trouble-free.

Week-by-week guide

Week One

You've chosen your diet days and your menu plan. You've read up on what you can and cannot eat. You're ready and raring to go. So let's get started.

Week 1, day 1 is probably going to be your hardest. It is the day when you have to be strictest about counting calories and the day you are likely to feel the hungriest. Yet it is also the day when you are most motivated. Think positively and just remember you only have to experience it once and you will find day 2 much easier. Just think of the all the lovely food you can eat tomorrow and maybe check if your stomach is just a little bit flatter.

You may also be able to get on the scales the morning after your first fasting day and see a drop of a pound or two. How's that for motivation?

In your first week, you should be very aware of what you are eating and when you eat.

Make the most of the calories you can eat and eat things that will fill you up for longer with the least amount of calories. This generally means eating mainly proteins – eggs, chicken or fish – with plenty of vegetables and salad. Carbohydrates like bread, pasta and rice contain lots of calories and you will burn up the energy and be hungry again quickly afterwards.

Beware of what you drink. There are plenty of no calorie or low calorie drinks out there. Water, diet colas, black tea or coffee are all fine. But drinks with milk add calories and a simple glass of orange juice could have nearly 100 calories.

Check the labels on everything you eat. Most food bought from supermarkets now has an exact calorie count for each item. This will be more accurate than the necessarily more general advice given here. Get your calculator out and add in every little thing.

The easiest way to follow the 5:2 diet in the first week is to stick to a menu plan. Remember that you can adapt the examples given here if you find it easier to eat at different times or if you've got different things in your cupboard.

Take it easy and even try and enjoy it. Relish your non-diet days and congratulate yourself at the end of each diet day.

Benefits you are likely to see in the first week

If you've made it through the first two days of fasting then you should be congratulating yourself. The next week's fasting days will be so much easier. Benefits such as increased energy are coming soon. But the thing you'll notice first will be weight-loss. You will be at your lightest before you eat at the start of the day following the second fast day. How much you lose will be determined by your starting weight and your body type. But some weight-loss is pretty much guaranteed.

Week Two

In Week 2 you should follow an almost identical pattern to week 1 but you will find it significantly easier.

Week 2 is all about building on week 1 and getting your body used to fasting. You should find the hunger pangs are less frequent and milder.

Weeks Three and Four

In weeks 3 and 4 your diet days are no longer a shock to the system. As your body is now used to the diet it should be getting significantly easier. You are unlikely to feel light-headed or grumpy during the day as your body is now finding the diet more natural.

In fact, the human body is not particularly designed for a regular daily calorie intake; this is a more modern invention. Back in the days of hunter-gatherers good meals were infrequent and they necessarily only ate by feast and famine. Our bodies are still built to cope well with this and the 5:2 diet is just trying to adapt the body back to this state.

If you've been following one of the menu plans then you finish your plan at the end of week 3. There's nothing to stop you starting again at the beginning in week 4, but now is the time that you'll probably want to adapt the diet a little to suit your needs. You'll be feeling more comfortable about how the 5:2 works and have found some recipes that you like and that fit your lifestyle. If there's any particular aspect of the menu plan you found hard it's worth trying out one of the other plans and seeing if it suits you better.

Mainly you should still consider the menu plan your guide; feel free to branch out, try some other recipes and generally make the 5:2 diet your own.

Benefits you are likely to see in the first month

As you near the end of your first month of 5:2 dieting you will find that your body has adapted fully to this diet as a way of life. I hope that you can begin to enjoy your fasting days and to feel healthier in body and spirit.

As well as continuing to lose weight (and doesn't that feel good!) you may well notice an increase in energy. Contrary to what you might expect on a diet day you feel energised and ready for anything.

Also, under the hood and hard to measure, the longer-term health benefits should be starting to kick in. If you started with raised cholesterol levels they may have started to drop. And even though you might not be able to see them outwardly some of those longer term, age-related health risks will now be reducing.

Into the future

If you've made it this far then all you need to do is carry on in exactly the same way and continue to reap the benefits. The 5:2 diet is not a fad; you should find it easy to carry it on for years to come. More than that you should want to keep doing it because it's so simple to follow and the benefits are so amazing.

By all means take a break for Christmas or when you go on holiday, you deserve it. And you know that you can just kick back into the diet when you get back and those holiday pounds will soon disappear.

I hope that above all you can see the 5:2 diet positively as something that you can continue. To many people who start down this route it is not a diet; it is a way of life that allows them to maintain a healthy weight while eating what they want. And according to research they are gaining great long term health benefits too.

Extending your weight-loss

If you have found that your weight-loss has slowed down and you feel like you need a little extra diet boost you could consider an occasional extra diet day or adding in gentle exercise on a diet day.

Low intensity exercise

Add half an hour of low intensity exercise such as walking, swimming or a light gym session on your fasting days.

Choose whatever exercise suits you best; it can be as simple as a gentle walk. You can fit the exercise in whenever you like during the day. A particularly nice time to exercise is in the evening as you will have less time to feel hungry afterwards and it's often a nice way to end the day. The most important thing to remember is not to push yourself as you won't have as much strength as on a normal day. Note that you can carry on exercising as normal (or not) on your feast days.

Exercise adds the following advantages to your 5:2 diet:

- improves your body shape and tone more than exercising on your feast days
- increases your weight-loss
- gives you more vitality
- distraction from hunger pangs
- exercise is less punishing and more fun

Occasional third diet day

If the 5:2 fasting is continuing to work well for you then this option is not for you. You should only consider fasting an extra day if you have been successfully following the 5:2 diet for at least six weeks and are finding that your body has fully adjusted to fasting days. This does not add to the health benefits of fasting but can give your weight-loss a boost.

Adding a third fast day in a week could be considered when one or more of the following are true:

- you have reached a weight-loss plateau
- you are preparing for a party or event and want to look your best the next day
- as a pre-emptive measure – you have a big party or event ahead of you and you want to be able to eat and drink more than normal without the usual guilt

The rules for a third day of fasting are effectively the same as for the other fasting days. You must have a feast day between each fast day.

I would not advise this as a normal course of events. I would advise it only occasionally, say once a month at most to have the most effect.

Personally I find a third fast day rather hard to fit into my normal routine and only do it very rarely. What I have found works well for me instead is an extra half day.

2 ½ fast days and 4 ½ feast days

It's not exactly a good name for a diet is it? This is something I follow more often than not as it fits practically into my life. Let me explain.

When I am thinking about which days to fast each week I normally reach the following conclusion:

I don't want to fast at the weekend. Therefore, Monday is an obvious fast day. I know this is the choice of the majority of 5:2 dieters. Tuesday must then be a feast day which leaves Wednesday or Thursday for fasting. If Wednesday fits suitably into my calendar I tend to go for Wednesday. Which means if I want to add an extra fast day into my week then it would need to be on Friday. BUT I have a problem with Fridays. On Friday's I might want to go out in the evening and if not I'll be most likely wanting a relaxing glass of wine at home to celebrate the start of the weekend.

I think more than one of you reading this must have reached a similar conclusion. So I have found a third option for ultimate weight-loss that does not rule out any of my normal treats.

Monday: fast day, 500 (650 for men) calories

Tuesday: feast day

Wednesday: fast day, 500 (650 for men) calories

Thursday: feast day

Friday: **fast day until 6pm**

On Friday (or whichever day you choose for a half-day fast) you should follow normal fasting rules until 6pm and then anything goes. So you would have your standard meagre breakfast on Friday and then fast until 6pm. But at 6pm you can eat normally and no longer count calories. This works because the fast is long enough to shake your body into fasting mode. Also, it is hard to eat a full day's worth of calories in the evening. I estimate that even with pizza, wine and biscuits (a typical Friday evening in our house!) my calorie count for the half day is about 1000 calories. But I don't calorie count on the Friday; I just enjoy my evening as well-earned and am all set for a relaxing and fun weekend.

Maintaining your weight

What if you've been following the 5:2 diet for a while and you are now at your target weight? Do you want to continue to have the health benefits of the 5:2 diet but you don't want to actually lose any more weight?

The simple answer is to cut back your fasting days to one a week. This is maintenance mode and you shouldn't lose weight with only fasting one day a week. If you continue to lose weight you could always stop altogether for a month or so and then do occasional fasting days.

We don't know whether one day a week of calorie restriction is enough to get all the health benefits, but in as much as we do know today it is likely that you will continue to cut your risk factors for age-related diseases.

How the 5:2 diet can help you live longer

So what about the amazing health benefits of which we've seen such tantalizing glimpses? A healthy long-life and a lower risk of heart disease, cancer and Alzheimer's. If this is all true then surely everyone would be on this diet?

Until very recently fasting was considered one of the more extreme dieting options; shunned by the mainstream medical profession as dangerous. It is only with this new breed of short non-total fasts, of which the 5:2 diet is the most popular and the easiest, that intermittent fasting is becoming more recognised as an option.

As a result research into short-term fasting is still in its infancy. At present we have a small selection of interesting studies from both sides of the Atlantic which have all produced some encouraging results. We have Professor Longo in California, who has been investigating the effects of the growth hormone IGF-1; research at Manchester University into the reduction of cancer risks; studies at Newcastle University into reversal of Type 2 diabetes through fasting; Krista Varady's research in Chicago into reducing the risk factors of heart disease; and research in Baltimore into how the 5:2 diet may protect us against brain diseases such as Alzheimer's.

We should do well to remember that as yet there are no long-term studies into the results of intermittent fasting; for this we have to look into the past and learn from history and some of the great world religions.

Professor Valter Longo at the Longevity Institute at the University of Southern California has been investigating insulin-like growth factor 1 (known as IGF-1), a hormone produced in the liver which keeps our cells growing.

When we eat normally our cells are constantly active and grow too fast for damage to be repaired effectively. When we fast levels of IGF-1 drop and we enter a state known as "autophagy" where our bodies produce less new cells and concentrate on repairing old ones. This effectively slows the ageing process while we fast.

Professor Longo has been working with Laron mice, which have been genetically engineered so that they don't respond to IGF-1. These mice are very small and exceptionally long-lived. They can live for up to five years which is more than twice the expected life-span of a normal mouse. In human terms that's equivalent to living to as much as 160 years old. Additionally these mice are pretty much immune to heart disease and cancer, and simply die of old age when their time comes.

Longo has also studied villagers from a remote community in Ecuador who have a genetic defect known as Laron syndrome. This is incredibly rare, affecting less than 350 people world-wide. People with Laron syndrome are short (less than 4ft tall) and, like the Laron mice, do not respond to IGF-1. They are also long-lived (although not exceptionally so). Most interestingly of all they appear to be resistant to cancer, diabetes and heart disease; there is not a single known case of someone with Laron syndrome dying of cancer.

The research by Professor Longo has shown that fasting lowers levels of IGF-1 and switches on DNA repair genes. Simply put, when our bodies run out of food our cells change from "growth" to "repair" mode.

Another study, this time from the National Institute on Ageing in Baltimore, has shown that reducing your calorie intake two days a week (i.e. the 5:2 diet) may protect against Alzheimer's, Parkinson's and other degenerative brain conditions. Professor Mark Mattson, who has led the study at the institute's laboratory of neurosciences, says that he and his colleagues have worked out a mechanism by which the growth of neurones in the brain could be affected by reduced calorie intakes. Intermittent fasting increases nerve cell growth factor which in turn protects neurons in the brain against the adversities of ageing. This may well reduce the risk factors for cognitive diseases such as Alzheimer's.

Mattson insists there are evolutionary reasons for believing it to be the case. "When resources became scarce, our ancestors would have had to scrounge for food," said Mattson. "Those whose brains responded best – who remembered where promising sources of food could be found or recalled how to avoid predators – would have been the ones who got the food. Thus a mechanism linking periods of starvation to neural growth would have evolved."

As we have seen in other studies this research is still in it's early stages, with human studies only just beginning.

In the UK a study by researchers at Newcastle University into the effects of fasting on sufferers of Type 2 diabetes has had some incredible results. In an early stage clinical trial all 11 volunteers reversed their diabetes by drastically cutting their food intake to just 600 calories a day for two months. And three months after the diet finished 70% remained free of diabetes. Professor Roy Taylor of Newcastle University who led the study said: "To have people free of diabetes after years with the condition is remarkable – and all because of an eight week diet."

Participants on the study found the diet very, very difficult to stick to and were only able to do so with the close supervision of a medical team. But for these volunteers the results were astonishing. Most were taking diabetes medicine before the trial and at the end found their insulin levels to be normal and that they no longer needed their medication.

Also in the UK, this time at the University of Manchester, a study of women following a strict 650 calorie diet just two days a week were found to lower their risk of breast cancer by 40%. The study, led by Dr Michelle Harvie, examined 50 overweight women from Greater Manchester. After six months following a 650-calorie-a-day diet for two days a week (and eating normally the rest of the week) the women had dropped an average of 13lb and showed major improvements in key areas linked to breast cancer. The women found their levels of the hormone leptin (known as a cancer risk factor) dropped 40% and their insulin levels dropped by up to 25%. Pamela Goldberg, chief executive of the Breast Cancer Campaign, said "This intermittent dieting approach provides an alternative to conventional dieting which could help with weight loss, but also potentially reduce the risk of developing breast cancer."

Finally, and perhaps the most relevant study, is on-going research by Dr Krista Varady at the University of Illinois at Chicago. Dr Varady has been studying a diet known as ADF, Alternate Day Fasting, where you eat restricted calories (600 for a man, 500 for a woman) every other day. The

5:2 diet is a less dramatic variant of the same diet. Dr Varady's research has three main aims: to find a diet that people can stick to for long periods of time, to see what weight-loss can be expected when following ADF for up to a year and to study the effect of intermittent fasting on certain heart disease risk factors, such as cholesterol and blood pressure.

As the study is still progressing the final conclusion is unavailable. Initial results are promising, however, with a low drop-out rate, gradual and continued weight-loss in most subjects and some impressive falls in cholesterol (down 21%), LDL ("bad") cholesterol (down 25%) and blood pressure.

Another interesting trial from Dr Varady took two groups of volunteers doing ADF for 10 weeks. One group were put on a low-fat diet on their feast days, while the other were encouraged to eat a typical high-fat American diet. Everyone, including Dr Varady, expected that the high-fat group would lose less weight than those following the low-fat diet. But they didn't, people on the high-fat diet were losing as much and sometimes even more weight, week after week. This suggests that we can eat what we want on our non-diet days as it really makes no difference.

The recipes

This is a book of ideas for eating healthy, well-balanced and low calorie food, perfect for the days when you have to watch your calories.

Every recipe here is specifically designed to keep you feeling satisfied for longer. This is done by choosing lean proteins, low fats and complex carbohydrates and combining them with bold flavours. Although a few recipes require a smaller portion size most provide you with a healthy "normal" plate of food.

The majority of recipes are for one portion but could be doubled up. Where this isn't practical the recipe makes two servings, suitable for sharing with your partner or keeping for another day. There are also plenty of recipes that are suitable to serve to your family.

The recipes include some practical suggestions for making larger quantities for freezing so you have a selection of your own ready meals to choose from. You can then take a portion to work or have one ready when you get home with a minimal amount of fuss.

Finally, everything is simple to prepare and cook. The ingredients are all readily available in any supermarket. There's nothing too fancy or expensive here.

So please use this as an inspiration and a starting point for your own 5:2 cooking. Just because you're on a diet (for 1 day!) doesn't mean you have to be hungry...

Breakfast ideas

Under 100 calories

A perfect Caffé Latte at home
37 calories per cup

Serves 1 Cook time: 3m

100ml skimmed milk
1 generous scoop or tablespoon of good quality ground coffee
100ml boiling water
Cafetière or other coffee brewing device

Pour 100ml boiling water over your coffee. Leave to brew for 2 minutes. Meanwhile heat 100ml skimmed milk until it is warm. Too hot and it will form a skin. You can do this on the hob until it gives off the first hint of steam or by giving it approximately 40 seconds in the microwave on high. When the coffee has brewed for two minutes plunge the cafetière and pour into the warm milk. Make sure you get the last dregs of the coffee as this gives it its froth. Now get the coffee back up to temp by giving it another microwave blast of about 30 seconds.

Blackberry fool
45 calories per serving

Serves 1 Prep time: 2m

50g blackberries
50g 0% fat Greek yoghurt

Mush the blackberries slightly with a fork and fold in the Greek yoghurt.

Egg white omelette
57 calories per serving

Serves 1 Prep time: 2m Cook time: 2m

3 large eggs
3 sprays light sunflower oil

First separate your eggs. Have 2 bowls in front of you. Crack the egg on the side of one of the bowls. Holding the egg over one of the bowls tip the egg yolk from one half of the shell to the other, letting the egg white drip out into the bowl below. Keep tipping the yolk from one half of the shell to the other until all the white is in the bowl. Then put the yolk in the second bowl. Repeat for the other 2 eggs. Whisk the egg whites together using a fork.

Spray your oil into a wide pan and heat on a medium setting for at least 2 minutes. Then add your egg whites. Sprinkle on plenty of salt and pepper. The omelette should cook in less than a minute. Serve immediately.

Natural yoghurt with kiwi
91 calories per serving

Serves 1 Prep time: 2m

100g low fat natural yoghurt
1 kiwi

Remove the skin from the kiwi and dice really small. Place in a bowl and mush lightly with a fork. Stir in the yoghurt.

Hot chocolate
102 calories per serving

Serves 1 Cook time: 2m

200ml skimmed milk
1 tsp cocoa
1 tsp sugar

Heat the milk gently on the hob until lightly steaming or in the microwave for approximately one minute. Stir in the cocoa and sugar.

Under 150 calories

Porridge pot
126 calories per serving

Porridge is a lovely warming and filling breakfast. This is a porridge pot because it's about half of a normal serving. Serve in a small dish such as a ramekin.

Serves 1 Cook time: 3m

20g rolled porridge oats
150ml skimmed milk

In a large bowl or measuring jug stir the milk into the oats. Heat in the microwave on high for two minutes. Consistency is everything with porridge; it should be thick without being gelatinous and liquid without being runny. If it's too thick add in some more milk a little at a time while stirring. If it's too thin, stir and microwave for another 30 seconds.

Under 200 calories

Baked beans on toast
172 calories per serving

Hardly a proper recipe but this is very warming and filling. Sometimes you can't beat beans on toast.

Serves 1 Cook time: 3m

1 slice reduced calorie wholemeal or granary bread
50g (¼ standard 415g can) reduced sugar and salt beans

Warm the beans and pour over the toast!

Healthy fry up
178 calories per serving

This isn't going to compete with a traditional fry up in terms of taste (and calories) but it is healthy, filling and delicious.

Serves 1 Cook time: 10m

2 reduced fat bacon rashers
1 large egg
1 tomato, chopped in half
3 sprays light sunflower oil spray

Heat a large frying pan on a medium heat for 2 minutes before adding the ingredients. Spray 3 squirts of light oil spray into the pan to prevent sticking. Add the bacon and the two tomato halves to the pan. Fry for about 3 minutes until they are both starting to brown on one side. Then turn the bacon and tomatoes over, leaving room for the egg. Crack the egg into the pan as well. Fry for another three minutes and then serve immediately.

Healthy fry up with baked beans
194 calories per serving

An alternative fry up which makes use of the ultra sustaining qualities of baked beans.

Serves 1 Cook time: 10m

1 reduced fat bacon rasher
1 large egg
50g (¼ standard 415g can) reduced sugar and salt baked beans
3 sprays light sunflower oil spray

Heat a large frying pan on a medium heat for 2 minutes. Spray 3 squirts of light oil spray into the pan. Add the bacon to the pan. Fry for about 3 minutes before turning and adding the egg. Fry for another 3 minutes. Heat the beans in a small saucepan or in a bowl in the microwave for 1 minute (30 seconds, stir, 30 seconds). Serve immediately.

Home-made granola
199 calories per serving (inc. 100ml skimmed milk)

Serves 8 Prep time: 10m Cook time: 15m

120g rolled oats
1 tbsp pumpkin seeds
1 tbsp sunflower seeds
40g pistachios, shelled and chopped
40g chopped hazelnuts
juice of 1 lemon
1 tbsp honey
40g raisins

Mix the oats, seeds and nuts together in a bowl. Stir together the lemon juice and honey and add to the dry ingredients, mixing well.

Spread evenly over a large baking sheet and bake in a pre-heated oven at 180C (160C fan, 360F) for 10 minutes. Add the raisins to the baking sheet and bake for a further 5 minutes. When cool can be stored in an airtight container for up to 2 weeks. Serve with 100ml of skimmed milk.

Under 300 calories

Scrambled eggs with peppers and tomatoes
249 calories per serving

Originally from the Basque region of France, this is scrambled eggs like you've never seen them before.

Serves 1 Prep time: 5m Cook time: 15m

1 tsp olive oil
½ onion, finely diced
1 clove garlic, sliced
1 red pepper, de-seeded and diced
½ tin tomatoes, chopped
1 large egg
1 egg white (see egg white omelette for instructions on how to separate an egg)
3 fresh basil leaves if you have them

Heat the oil in a frying pan and add the onions, garlic and peppers. Fry them gently on a medium heat for 8 minutes, until golden. Tip in the chopped tomatoes and cook for another 5 minutes.

Meanwhile, whisk together the egg and egg white and season with salt and pepper. Pour the eggs into the frying pan with the other ingredients, stirring constantly until they thicken like scrambled eggs – about 3 minutes. Serve with basil on the top.

Salads

Under 100 calories

Standard salad
78 calories per serving (including salad dressing)

A lot of the recipes listed later on call for a salad as an accompaniment. Here is what I would put into a standard salad for one person, totalling 68 cals per portion.

Serves 1 Prep time: 5m

¼ *iceberg lettuce*
2 *inches* cucumber
2 *medium* tomatoes

Using a serving (1 tablespoon) of pre-bought light salad dressing will add approximately 10 calories.

"German" salad
94 calories per serving (including salad dressing)

Add a little variety to your salads...

Serves 1 Prep time: 5m

¼ *iceberg lettuce*
2 *inches* cucumber
2 *medium* tomatoes
2 *large* or 3 *small* gherkins
2 *tsp* capers
1 *tbsp* light salad dressing

Ham or bacon salad
98 calories per serving

A little bit more filling than a standard salad.

¼ iceberg lettuce
2 inches cucumber
1 medium tomato
1 slice of ham or 1 low fat bacon rasher
1 tbsp light salad dressing

Under 200 calories

Chargrilled vegetable salad
127 calories per serving

You prepare this salad by grilling the vegetables and then marinating overnight. Ideal for preparing the night before and taking to work the next day.

Serves 2 Prep time: 10m Cook time: 10m Marinate time: 8h

4 sprays light oil spray
1 small aubergine, sliced widthways into thin slices
1 courgette, sliced lengthways thinly
4 spring onions
1 red pepper, de-seeded and quartered
6 asparagus spears

½ shallot, diced
½ red chilli, de-seeded and finely sliced
1 clove garlic, sliced
4 basil leaves, shredded
1 tbsp extra virgin òlive oil
2 tsp red wine vinegar

Use a griddle pan if you've got one or a normal frying pan would do fine. Spray the pan with the 4 sprays of oil and heat to a moderate heat. Grill all the vegetables for about 10 minutes, turning once. You may need to do this in two separate batches.

Combine the diced shallot, chilli, garlic, basil, oil and vinegar in a dish and toss over the vegetables while they are still warm. Make sure all the vegetables are covered in the marinade before leaving overnight to marinate. Serve at room temperature.

Oriental prawn and mushroom salad
151 calories per serving

Serves 1 Prep time: 5m

60g chestnut mushrooms, washed and finely sliced
75g jumbo prawns, cooked
50g baby spinach or other salad leaves
1 spring onion, sliced
2 tsp rice vinegar
juice ½ lemon
1 tsp light soy sauce
1 tsp olive oil

Cut the prawns in half and combine with the mushrooms, spring onion and salad leaves. In a small bowl mix together the rice vinegar, lemon juice, soy sauce and olive oil. Pour the dressing over the salad and toss well.

Italian bread salad
170 calories per serving

Serves 1 Prep time: 5m Marinate time: 30m

½ thick slice granary bread
6 ripe cherry tomatoes, quartered
1 spring onion, sliced
2 inches cucumber, diced
½ clove garlic, crushed
2 basil leaves, shredded
1 tsp extra virgin olive oil
2 tsp red wine vinegar

This salad is best if the bread is not fresh. Remove the crust from the bread and cut into chunks. Place the bread in a bowl and sprinkle with a little water. Add the tomatoes, spring onion, cucumber and celery and mix gently. In a small bowl mix together the garlic, basil, olive oil and red wine vinegar to make the dressing and pour over the salad. Leave for half an hour at room temperature for the flavours to develop.

Warm bean salad
199 calories per serving

Serves 1 Prep time: 2m Cook time: 4m

⅓ can mixed beans, drained (90g)
80g green beans, fresh or frozen
2 tsp extra virgin olive oil
juice of ½ lemon
salt and pepper

Place the mixed beans in a small saucepan and add just enough water to cover them. Warm through on a medium heat for 5 minutes. Meanwhile boil your green beans for 3 minutes. Drain both your mixed beans and your green beans and place in a bowl. While still warm mix in the oil, lemon juice and seasoning.

Under 300 calories

Prawn, wild rice and rocket salad
211 calories per serving

Serves 1 Cook time: 30m Prep time: 2m

30g red or wild rice
75g prawns, cooked (if frozen, defrosted)
50g rocket leaves
juice of ½ lemon
½ tsp extra virgin olive oil
freshly ground black pepper

Cook the rice in boiling water for 30 minutes, or as per pack instructions if different. Leave to cool. In a bowl mix together the rice and rocket and then place the prawns on the top. Squeeze over the lemon juice and a small drizzle (½ teaspoon) of olive oil. Finally sprinkle on a little black pepper.

Salade Nicoise
292 calories per serving

A classic; substantial and tasty.

Serves 1 Prep time: 10m

1 little gem lettuce, separated into leaves
1 tomato, quartered
1 hard-boiled egg, cut into quarters
40g green beans, cooked (from fresh or frozen)
½ can tuna in water or brine (185g)
1 anchovy fillet, dried on kitchen paper
5 black olives

For the dressing:
1 tsp extra virgin olive oil
1 tsp white wine vinegar
1 tsp capers
salt and pepper

Mix together the dressing ingredients and set aside. Place the lettuce leaves in a bowl and add the tomato, green beans and hard-boiled egg. Roughly flake the tuna and add in. Pour the dressing over the salad. Top with the anchovy fillet and scatter over the olives.

Egyptian chicken salad
293 calories per serving

Serves 2 Prep time: 10m

2 chicken breasts, cooked (approx 340g)
3 inches cucumber, roughly cubed
10 cherry tomatoes, halved
½ red pepper, diced
2 spring onions, finely chopped
4 mint leaves, shredded
4 parsley leaves, shredded
2 little gem lettuces, shredded

For the dressing:
2 tsp extra virgin olive oil
juice of 1 lemon
½ clove garlic, finely chopped
1 tsp ground cumin
salt and pepper

Mix together the dressing ingredients in a small cup or bowl and set aside to rest for 5 minutes. Place the chicken, cucumber, tomatoes, red pepper, spring onions, lettuce and herbs in another large bowl and toss the dressing over, making sure everything is well-coated.

Warm leek and lentil salad with goat's cheese
298 calories per serving

This is an extremely filling and warming dish.

Serves 1 Prep time: 5m Soak time: 15m Cook time: 30m

50g puy lentils (dry weight)
2 leeks
2 sprays light sunflower oil
½ clove garlic, finely chopped
5 sun-dried tomatoes
30g light feta/Greek style cheese
few drops balsamic vinegar

Put the dried tomatoes in a small cup. Pour in boiling water so the cup is about ¼ full. Leave to soak. Wash the lentils under running water for a minute before transferring to a small saucepan and covering with about 2cm cold water. Bring up to the boil and simmer gently for 25 minutes until cooked. Top up with more water if it starts to look dry.

Meanwhile chop your leeks finely. In a wide saucepan with a lid, add a few sprays of light oil and when at a medium heat add the leeks and garlic and fry for 3-4 minutes. As the leeks start to brown add half a cup of water, stir and put the lid on the pan. Cook for another 6 minutes. Chop the feta into very small squares. Remove the tomatoes from their soaking liquid and cut into small pieces. Stir the tomatoes and lentils into the leeks. Place in a bowl and top with the feta and a drizzle of balsamic vinegar.

Light lunches

As you may well have already found the nation's lunch-time staple, bread (in all its many forms), contains a substantial number of calories. Most of the lunch choices in this section contain bread, pitta or flatbread because that is what we enjoy and find convenient for our lunch-time meal. However, we need to make clever choices to ensure the meal does not contain too many calories. To do this it is easiest to buy reduced calorie bread products which have clear labelling on the number of calories per slice. I only ever use bread products that you can buy from any supermarket. Here are some of the best that I have found:

Warburtons Thins, plain or seeded (100 calories)

These are small rolls or flatbreads that come pre-cut into halves. They can used as a normal roll, toasted or used to make an open sandwich.

German style rye bread (101 calories per slice)

A filling and tasty alternative to bread. One of my favourite lunch-time snacks is pastrami on rye.

Oatcakes (47 calories per oatcake)

Low calorie tortilla wraps (130 calories)

Pitta bread (160 calories)

Under 150 calories

Oatcake with peanut butter and tomato
97 calories per serving

This is a favourite snack of mine. My husband thinks I'm weird, but I find the tomato takes off the sometimes cloying edge of the peanut butter and the balsamic gives it an extra zing.

Serves 1 Preparation time: 2m

1 oatcake
1 tsp peanut butter
1 slice tomato
few drops of balsamic vinegar

Spread the peanut butter evenly over the oatcake and top with the slice of tomato. Drizzle a little balsamic over the top.

Rye bread with soft cheese and cucumber
132 calories per serving

Serves 1 Prep time: 2m

1 slice rye bread
20g light soft cheese (about 1 tbsp)
4 thick slices cucumber

Cut the rye bread into quarters. Spread an even quantity of soft cheese on each quarter and top with a slice of cucumber. Season with salt and pepper.

Pastrami on rye
137 calories per serving

An American mustard such as French's is great here. But English mustard also works well.

Serves 1 Preparation time: 5m

1 slice rye bread
1 tsp American or English mustard
2 slices pastrami
4 small/ 2 large gherkins in sweet vinegar

Spread the mustard thinly over the rye bread and cut it in half. Place one slice of pastrami on each half of the bread. Slice the gherkins extremely thinly lengthways. Lay the gherkins evenly over the pastrami.

Home-made salsa on flatbread
144 calories per serving

The best flatbreads I have found are "Warburtons thins", available from supermarkets but any diet bread that is 100 calories per slice would be perfectly suitable.

Salsa serves 4 Prep time: 10m Infuse time: 1h

¼ red onion
1 green chilli, de-seeded
1 spring onion
1 clove garlic
4 tomatoes
1 tsp olive oil
½ to 1 tsp salt
juice of 1 lemon
1 tsp tomato purée
1 tbsp water
1 flatbread

Combine the red onion, green chilli, spring onion and garlic in a food processor. Whizz until finely chopped. Add the tomatoes (whole, with skins and seeds all ok!), olive oil, salt, lemon juice, tomato purée and water. Pulse the food processor until just chopped; you want it chunky. Transfer to a bowl and check the salt. Leave for ½ to 1 hour for the flavours to infuse.

Serve by spreading ¼ of the mix generously over a toasted flatbread.

Under 200 calories

Smoked salmon and cream cheese on oatcakes
169 calories per serving

Serves 1 Prep time: 5m

2 oatcakes
2 tsp low fat cream cheese
1 slice smoked salmon (20g)
1 slice lemon
freshly ground black pepper

Spread 1 teaspoon of cream cheese over both oatcakes. Cut the piece of salmon in two and put one on each oatcake. Top with a blob (½ teaspoon) of cream cheese. Squeeze on a little lemon juice and add a sprinkling of black pepper.

BLT flatbread
173 calories per serving

You won't feel like you're dieting if you have one of these!

Prep time: 2m Cook time: 5m

1 low cal flatbread
1 low fat/diet bacon rasher
1 tsp lighter mayonnaise
1 medium tomato, sliced
finely sliced lettuce

Grill or dry fry the bacon as per the instructions. Lightly toast the flatbread.

Spread the mayonnaise thinly over the flatbread and top with the lettuce.

Put the bacon rasher on next and finally add the sliced tomato.

Rye bread with taramasalata
195 calories per serving

Serves 1 Prep time: 2m

1 slice rye bread
20g good quality shop-bought taramasalata

Cut the rye bread into 8 pieces and spread a little taramasalata over each one. Sprinkle with a tiny bit of black pepper.

Easy houmous with vegetables for dipping
195 calories per serving

Makes 8 servings of houmous (139 calories per serving)

Prep time: 10m

1 can chick peas
5 tbsp tahini paste (90g)
2 cloves garlic, peeled
juice of 2 lemons
2 tbsp olive oil
pinch cayenne pepper
salt and pepper

For dipping per person:
½ red pepper, de-seeded and sliced into batons
2 inches cucumber, cut into batons
½ carrot, peeled and cut into batons

Blitz the chick peas and garlic in a food processor with a little water from the can until smooth. Add the tahini, lemon juice, cayenne pepper and a good pinch of salt and pepper. Blitz again until really smooth. Turn into a dish or individual portions. Can keep for up to 3 days in the fridge. Serve an individual portion in a small dish or ramekin, surrounded by the vegetable batons.

Ham omelette
198 calories per serving

You probably don't need instructions for this, but I've included them just in case.

Serves 1 Prep time: 2m Cook time:3m

2 large eggs
1/2 slice ham, cut into small pieces
4 sprays of sunflower oil spray such as Fry Light

Put the eggs and a tablespoon of water in a bowl. Whisk the eggs together using a fork. Pour them into a hot, oiled frying pan, making sure they cover the bottom. After about 30 seconds lift up one side of the omelette with a wooden spoon and tilt the pan slightly to allow some of the uncooked egg to fill the gap. Repeat all around the omelette until it no longer runs. Spread the ham evenly over the top. Give it another 30 seconds before folding and sliding onto a plate.

Cucumber dip with home-made tortilla chips
200 calories per serving

Serves 2 Prep time: 5m Infuse time: 30m Cook time: 5m

150g 0% fat natural yoghurt
2 inches cucumber
2 tsp dried mint
pinch of salt
1 tsp extra virgin olive oil
2 low calorie tortilla wraps

Peel and coarsely grate the cucumber. Place in a small bowl with the yoghurt, mint and a pinch of salt. Stir well and leave for 30 minutes at room temperature for the flavours to develop.

Cut your wrap into small triangles and place on a non-stick baking tray. Pre-heat the oven to 220C (200F, 430F) and cook the tortilla chips for 4-5 minutes until golden brown. Remove from the oven and allow to cool on the baking tray, this will make them go crispy.

Place the dip in a serving dish and drizzle with the olive oil. Serve the tortilla chips on a plate surrounding the dip.

Under 300 calories

Watercress falafel
230 calories per serving

Serve on a bed of watercress with lemon wedges on the side.

Serves 2 Prep time: 5m Cook time: 20m

1 can chickpeas, rinsed and drained
100g watercress
1 tablespoon tahini paste
1 clove garlic, peeled
juice ½ lemon
1 tsp baking powder
1 tsp cumin
½ tsp cayenne pepper
2 tsp olive oil

Place all the ingredients except the oil in a food processor and whizz until finely chopped but not puréed. Shape the mixture into 6 balls and flatten slightly with the palm of your hand. Brush the falafel with a little olive oil on both sides and arrange on a non-stick baking tray. Cook in a pre-heated oven at 200C (180C fan, 390F) for 18-20 minutes until golden brown.

Prawn in sweet chilli sauce wrap
239 calories per serving

Very simple to make, the sweet chilli sauce really adds a punch to this quick wrap.

Serves 1 Prep time: 2m

1 reduced calorie wrap
40g shredded iceberg lettuce (less than ¼)
75g prawns, cooked
1 tbsp sweet chilli dipping sauce

Put the prawns in a bowl with the chilli sauce and mix thoroughly. Spread your lettuce over the wrap, leaving 1 inch at the bottom free. Place your prawn mixture over the lettuce, making sure the prawns are near the middle but the sauce goes all over. Fold up the bottom inch and then roll carefully.

Roast chicken and pesto open flatbread
241 calories per serving

Serves 1 Prep time: 5m

60g ready-to-eat cooked roasted chicken (about ½ chicken breast)
2 tsp pesto
30g rocket leaves
1 low cal flatbread such as Warburtons thins

Spread 1 teaspoon of pesto thinly over both halves of the flatbread. Spread the rocket leaves evenly over that. Cut the chicken into bite size pieces and mix the remaining pesto into the chicken. Spread the pesto chicken over the flatbread and grind some black pepper over the top.

Feta salad on toasted flatbread
260 calories per serving

Serves 1 Prep time: 5m Cook time: 5m

30g reduced fat feta or Greek style cheese
1 tomato, diced
2 inches cucumber, diced
6 black olives pitted
2 basil leaves, torn
1 tsp extra virgin olive oil
1 tsp balsamic vinegar
freshly ground pepper
1 low cal flatbread such as Warburtons thins

Cut your feta into very small chunks and place in a bowl. Add in the tomato, cucumber and olives and mix. Toast your flatbread. Spread your salad equally over both slices of flatbread and drizzle over the olive oil and balsamic. Top with freshly ground pepper.

Refried beans and goat's cheese hot wrap
268 calories per serving

Serves 1 Prep time: 5m Cook time: 5m

1 reduced calorie wrap
¼ tin of kidney beans
few sprays light sunflower oil spray
few drops Worcestershire sauce
20g light goat's cheese
1 tomato
1 inch cucumber
juice of ½ lime

Put the kidney beans into a sieve and rinse. Using a fork gently press on the beans so they are broken up but not mashed.

Heat a small saucepan with the oil spray and add the kidney beans. Add salt and pepper and a few drops of Worcestershire sauce. Fry for about 5 minutes stirring occasionally until the beans start to go brown and crunchy.

Meanwhile prepare the goat's cheese salad. Chop the goat's cheese into very small cubes and place in a bowl. Cut the tomato and cucumber into small cubes and add to the bowl. Squeeze over the juice of the lime and stir in.

Heat the wrap in the microwave for 10 seconds. Lay it flat on a plate and spread the beans over the top, leaving an inch free at the bottom to fold over. Arrange the goat's cheese salad over the beans. Fold up the bottom inch and then roll up the wrap.

Chilli chicken pitta
273 calories per serving

Serves 1 Prep time: 5m Marinate time: 30m Cook time: 10m

2 spring onions, chopped finely
2 garlic cloves, chopped finely
juice ½ lemon
1 tsp honey
½ tsp paprika
¼ tsp mild chilli powder
½ chicken breast fillet
1 pitta bread
some iceberg lettuce

Mix together the spring onion, garlic, lemon juice, honey, paprika and chilli powder. Cut the chicken into small lumps, no bigger than 1 inch square. Stir the chicken into the lemony marinade. Leave for at least half an hour.

Turn up your grill to the highest setting and when hot put your chicken on your grill pan and cook for about 4 minutes each side. They should be brown and crispy all over.

Toast your pitta. Cut in half and stuff with the chicken and shredded lettuce.

Mexican five bean wrap
294 calories per serving

This is the most filling lunch you can imagine; you won't need to eat for the rest of the day after this. You can find ready-to-eat cans or pouches of 5 or 6 mixed beans (or mixed bean salad) in every supermarket.

Serves 1 Prep time: 5m

1 reduced calorie wrap
80g ready-to-eat mixed beans,drained (approx third of a can)
20g lighter cheddar
1 tbsp salsa
shredded lettuce

Rinse and drain the beans. Spread the salsa evenly over the whole wrap. Then add the beans, making sure you leave at least an inch free at the bottom of the wrap to fold over. Arrange your shredded lettuce over the beans and then grate over the cheese as evenly as possible. Fold over the bottom inch of the wrap. Then gently but firmly roll up the wrap.

Soups

All the soups listed here (with the exception of the Ramen soup) make four to six servings and can be frozen in individual portions.

Under 100 calories

Mushroom broth
44 calories per serving

Serves 4 Prep time: 5m Soak time: 10m Cook time: 30m

4 dried porcini mushrooms
250g chestnut mushrooms
1 litre vegetable or chicken stock, fresh is best here but if you need to use stock cubes you will need two
1 bay leaf
sprig fresh thyme
sprig fresh rosemary
3 leaves fresh parsley, chopped
3 tbsp sherry or Madeira (50ml)

Firstly, place the porcini mushrooms in a cup and cover with boiling water. Leave to reconstitute for 10 minutes. Prepare the chestnut mushrooms by washing and then slicing. Put the chestnut mushrooms and stock in a large saucepan and bring to simmering point. Remove the porcini mushrooms from their soaking liquid and chop finely. Add to the pan, together with the soaking liquid, discarding the gritty dregs. Add the fresh herbs and simmer gently for ½ hour. Add the sherry or Madeira just before serving.

Thai spinach soup
96 calories per serving

Serves 4 Prep time: 5m Cook time: 20m

1 tsp olive oil
1 medium onion, chopped
1 garlic clove, chopped
1 tsp ground cumin
1 litre vegetable stock, fresh or made with 2 stock cubes
1 tsp cornflour
100ml reduced fat coconut milk
250g fresh spinach
1 tbsp green Thai curry paste
juice 1 lime

Heat the oil gently in a large casserole dish and fry the onions and garlic for 5 minutes. Stir in the cumin and add the stock. Now cover, bring to the boil and simmer for 15 minutes.

Mix the cornflour with a little water and add to the simmering stock, stirring well. Stir in the coconut milk, lime juice and Thai curry paste until dissolved. Add in the spinach and cook for one minute. Transfer to a liquidiser and blend until smooth. Reheat gently in the pan.

Under 150 calories

Carrot and coriander soup
111 calories per serving

I think this is my favourite warming winter soup. I just wish I could get my children to like it!

Serves 4 Prep time: 10m Cook time: 45m

1 tbsp vegetable oil
1 large onion, sliced
500g/1lb carrots, peeled and sliced
1 tsp ground coriander
1¼ litres or 2 pints vegetable stock, fresh or made with 2 veg stock cubes
large bunch of fresh coriander, roughly chopped

Heat the oil gently in a large pan and add the onions and carrots. Cook for 5 minutes until starting to soften. Stir in the ground coriander and season with salt and pepper. Cook for a further minute. Add the vegetable stock and bring to the boil. Simmer for 40 minutes. Use a liquidiser to blend the soup until smooth. Reheat gently and stir in the fresh coriander just before serving.

Garlic soup
121 calories per serving

Garlic soup is very warming and hearty. It is also exceptionally good for you.

Serves 6 Prep time: 10m Cook time: 1h

2 large heads of garlic
2 onions
1 tbsp olive oil
1 tbsp cornflour
1½ litres or 2½ pints chicken/vegetable stock, either fresh or made with three chicken or veg stock cubes
1 tsp dried thyme
1 can of cannellini beans, rinsed and drained
1 tbsp red wine vinegar

Separate the cloves of garlic, peel and slice. Chop the onion. In a large heavy saucepan, cook the garlic and onions in the oil on a very gentle heat. Stir often and cook for about 10 minutes until the onions are translucent. Stir in the cornflour and thyme and then immediately start adding the stock. Add the stock gradually to avoid lumps. Bring to the boil and simmer for 45 minutes.

Transfer the soup to a liquidiser (in small batches) and blend until smooth. Return to the heat and add the beans and red wine vinegar. Warm through and serve with black pepper.

Lentil, lemon and thyme soup
121 calories per serving

An easy store cupboard soup

Makes 4 generous servings Prep time: 5m Cook time: 45m

1 tbsp olive oil
1 large onion, finely diced
1 garlic clove, finely chopped
150g red lentils, rinsed in a sieve
500ml vegetable stock, fresh or made from 1 stock cube
1 tin tomatoes, chopped
2 tsp tomato purée
2 tsp dried thyme, or 2 fresh sprigs
juice of ½ lemon

Heat the oil in a large saucepan and gently fry the onions and garlic for 5 minutes until soft. Add the lentils and stir into the onions. Pour in the stock, then bring to the boil. Simmer vigorously for 10 minutes. Reduce the heat and add the thyme, tinned tomatoes and purée. Bring back to a quiet simmer and simmer gently for 30 minutes. Add the lemon juice and season to taste.

Under 200 calories

Savoy cabbage and bacon soup
156 calories per serving

Serves 4 Prep time: 10m Cook time: 25m

1 tbsp olive oil
1 onion, roughly chopped
1 garlic clove, roughly chopped
1 medium potato, peeled and roughly chopped
600ml chicken stock, fresh or made with 1 stock cube
½ savoy cabbage, shredded
4 low fat bacon rashers, cut into strips
100ml reduced fat crème fraiche

Heat the oil in a large saucepan and gently fry the onions and garlic for 5 minutes. Add the potato and stock, bring to the boil and simmer for 10 minutes. Add the cabbage and cook for a further 5 minutes.

Transfer to a blender (possibly in two batches) and blend until smooth. Reheat the soup gently in the pan. In a separate frying pan dry fry the bacon strips until slightly brown on both sides (4-5 minutes). Stir the bacon and crème fraiche into the soup.

Pea and pesto soup
161 calories per serving

Serves 4 Prep time: 5m Cook time: 35m

1 tbsp olive oil
2 leeks, sliced
1 garlic clove, finely sliced
1 medium potato, peeled and diced
250g peas, fresh or frozen
500ml vegetable stock, fresh or made with 1 stock cube
50g broad beans, fresh or frozen
50g baby spinach leaves
1 tablespoon pesto

Heat the oil in a casserole or large saucepan and gently fry the leeks and garlic for 10 minutes. Add the potato, 200g of peas and the stock. Cover and simmer gently for 20 minutes.

Transfer the soup to a blender (possibly in two batches) and blend until smooth. Put the soup back in the pan and bring back to temperature. Stir in the peas, broad beans, spinach and pesto and season to taste. Bring to a gentle simmer and heat for a further 5 minutes.

Black-eyed beans and bacon soup
162 calories per serving

Serves 4 Prep time: 5m Cook time: 50m

4 low fat bacon rashers, cut into strips
1 can black-eyed beans, rinsed and drained
1 medium onion, finely chopped
1 medium carrot, finely chopped
1 stick celery, finely chopped
1 litre chicken stock, fresh or made with 2 stock cubes
2 cloves garlic, finely chopped
3 tbsp tomato purée
3 tsp chilli paste
1 tsp dried oregano

In a large casserole or saucepan dry fry the bacon strips for about 4 minutes until a little bit crispy. Then add the onion, carrot, celery, garlic and chicken stock, stir and bring to the boil. Add the rest of your ingredients: black-eyed beans, tomato puree, chilli paste and oregano and stir. Simmer gently for 45 minutes.

Spicy butternut squash soup
169 calories per serving

Serves 4 Prep time: 10m Cook time: 35m

1 tbsp olive oil
1 garlic clove, finely chopped
1 large or 2 small sweet potatoes (200g), peeled and diced
1 small butternut squash, peeled and diced
½ tsp smoked paprika
½ red chilli, de-seeded and chopped
750ml vegetable stock, fresh or made with 1 stock cube
1 tbsp wholegrain mustard
1 tbsp parmesan cheese, finely grated
100ml reduced fat crème fraiche

Heat the oil in a large casserole. Toss in the garlic, sweet potato and butternut squash. Stir, cover and cook gently for 10 minutes. Stir in the smoked paprika and red chilli. Add the stock and bring to the boil. Cover and simmer for 20 minutes.

Remove from the heat and stir in the mustard and parmesan.

Transfer to a blender in two batches and blend until smooth. Return the soup to the pan and add the crème fraiche. Reheat gently for 2 minutes and serve.

Chorizo and tomato soup
177 calories per serving

Makes 6 servings Prep time: 5m Cook time: 40m

1 tsp olive oil
1 onion, diced
1 garlic clove, finely sliced
1 green pepper, diced
100g chorizo, diced
500ml vegetable stock, fresh or made with one stock cube
1 tin tomatoes, chopped
300g passata
1 tin chick peas, rinsed and drained

Heat the oil in a saucepan, add the onion and cook gently for 5 minutes.

Add the garlic, green pepper and chorizo, then cook for a further 5 minutes.

Add the stock, tomatoes, passata and chick peas, then simmer for 30 minutes.

Red pepper soup with goat's cheese
192 calories per serving

Serves 6 Prep time: 10m Cook time: 35m

1 tbsp olive oil
1 large onion, roughly chopped
50g red lentils
1½ litres vegetable stock, made with 3 stock cubes
100ml white wine
8 red peppers, de-seeded and roughly chopped
1 large cooking apple, peeled, cored and chopped
2 tsp dried basil
150g rindless goat's cheese, roughly cut or broken up

Heat the olive oil gently in a large saucepan and fry the onions for 5 minutes. Add the lentils, stir and pour in half the stock. Bring to the boil and simmer vigorously for 10 minutes. Then add the red peppers, apple, basil, white wine and the rest of the stock. Bring back to a gentle simmer and cook for a further 30 minutes.

Transfer to a blender, you'll need to do this in two or more batches, and blend until smooth. Return the soup to the pan and reheat gently. Stir in the goat's cheese until melted, then serve.

Under 300 calories

Ramen soup with udon noodles
215 calories per serving

This soup is incredibly satisfying and warming and can be made in under 10 minutes.

Serves 1 Prep time: 5m Cook time: 5m

75g Udon wet noodles (¼ pack Sharwood's Udon wet noodles) or equivalent dry noodles cooked according to packet instructions
25g (heaped tablespoon) Miso soup paste
1 tsp mirin
1 tbsp dark soy sauce
½ inch fresh ginger, peeled and grated
50g spring greens or savoy cabbage, thinly sliced
½ carrot, cut into very fine batons
50g beansprouts
60g Shiitake mushrooms, washed and sliced

Bring 500ml water to boiling point in a saucepan. Stir in the miso paste, mirin, soy and ginger. Stir until the miso is dissolved. Add in the greens, carrot and mushrooms. Put the lid on the pan and simmer gently for 5 minutes.

In a separate pan pour boiling water over the noodles and simmer for 2 minutes. When they are warmed through drain and put them in a large soup bowl. Add the beansprouts to the ramen, stir and pour over the noodles. Drizzle a little good quality soy sauce over the top and serve.

Hearty ham soup
224 calories per serving

Two types of lentils plus the pearl barley make this a great recipe for a healthy heart.

Makes 4 servings Prep time: 10m Cook time: 1h 30m

1 tbsp olive oil
1 onion, finely diced
2 carrots, diced
30g red lentils
30g green puy lentils
30g pearl barley
750ml chicken stock, fresh or made with 1½ stock cubes
250g cooked ham or gammon, cut into bite sized pieces
1 medium potato, peeled and diced

Heat the oil in a large saucepan or casserole and fry the onions and carrots very gently for 10 minutes until the onions are transparent.

Rinse the lentils and pearl barley, stir into the pan and then add the stock. Bring to the boil, cover and simmer for 45 minutes. Add the ham and potato and simmer for a further 30 minutes.

Vegetables

Under 200 calories

Garlic mushrooms
107 calories per serving

Serves 1 Prep time: 5m Cook time: 10m

2 large flat mushrooms
2 tsp extra virgin olive oil
1 garlic clove, finely chopped
1 tsp fresh parsley, finely chopped

Prepare the mushrooms by cleaning off any soil and cutting out the stalks.
Cut the stalks up very small and mix in a small bowl with the oil, garlic and
parsley. Place the mushrooms top side up on a grill pan under a hot grill.
Grill for 4 minutes. Take out the grill pan and turn the mushrooms over.
Distribute the garlic and oil mixture evenly over the mushrooms. Sprinkle
with salt and pepper. Place back under the hot grill for a further 6 minutes.
Serve immediately.

Ratatouille
155 calories per serving

Serves 1 Prep time: 10m Salting time: 1h Cook time: 35m

1 small aubergine
1 courgette
1 tbsp salt
1 tsp olive oil
½ onion chopped
1 clove garlic chopped
½ red pepper, chopped
½ tin tomatoes
Some chopped fresh basil if you have it

(handwritten notes)
1 = 100gr =
1 = 150gr = 33 C
1 t =
½ = 90gr = 27.5 C
t = 50gr = 16 C
½ = 200gr = 42 C

(handwritten numbers in left margin: 4, 4, 4T, 4t, 2, 4, 2, 2)

Wash and slice the aubergine and courgette into ½ cm slices. Quarter the aubergine slices. Put the aubergines and courgettes into a colander over a bowl. Add the salt and place a plate on the top plus something to weigh it down. Leave for about an hour and you should get some brown bitter juice coming out of the bottom. Wash in cold water before cooking.

In a saucepan heat the olive oil and gently fry the onion and garlic for about 5 minutes. Add the chopped pepper and the aubergine and courgettes. Add basil if you have it and some salt and pepper. Put the lid on and turn the heat to low and cook for 20 minutes. Add the chopped tomatoes and heat gently for 10-15 minutes. Tastes even better if left to cool and then reheated.

Spinach and pea dahl
159 calories per serving

This is so tasty and filling that you really will forget you're on a diet.

Serves 4 Prep time: 10m Cook time: 50m

1 large onion
4 cloves garlic
1 inch thumb ginger
1 large red chilli
1 tbsp sunflower oil
½ pint red lentils
¼ tsp turmeric powder
¼ tsp cayenne pepper
1 tsp paprika
½ tsp ground cumin
1 tsp salt
2 pints water
1 tomato
juice of 1 lime
2 tbsp frozen peas
3 cubes frozen spinach

Put the oil in a heavy bottomed pan over a low to medium heat.

Peel and roughly chop (or pulse in a food processor) the onion, garlic and ginger. Then coarsely chop the chilli (removing the seeds and membrane if you don't want too much heat). Put all chopped ingredients into the pan and lightly fry until the onion starts to turn translucent (about 5 minutes).

Once the onion has softened add all the ground spices, stir well and fry for another minute or two.

Place the lentils in a sieve and rinse under the cold tap for a minute. Next add the lentils to the pan and give the mixture a really good stir before adding all the water and turning the heat right up. Get the water at a fierce boil for ten minutes before turning it right down again.

Now leave it on the lowest heat you can, stirring occasionally and watching that the dahl is not catching on the bottom of the pan. Over the next 30 to 45 minutes it will thicken up considerably. Keep stirring occasionally until you have the consistency of thick porridge. Then add spinach, peas, lime juice and roughly chopped tomato and cook for a further five minutes before serving.

Cauliflower curry
166 calories per serving

This curry is spicy but not hot.

Serves 2 Prep time: 10m Cook time: 25m

½ tsp ground cumin
½ tsp ground coriander
¼ tsp turmeric
1 tsp salt
juice ½ lemon
2 inch thumb fresh ginger, peeled and cut into matchsticks
1 tsp cumin seeds
½ tsp mustard seeds
1 tbsp groundnut oil
2 tomatoes, diced
1 medium sized cauliflower, cut into small florets

Firstly, mix all the ground spices and salt together in a small bowl. Add the lemon juice and 2 tbsp water.

In a large lidded frying pan heat the oil on a medium heat. Quickly stir in the ginger and fry for a minute before throwing in the cumin and mustard seeds. Cook for a minute and just as they start to sizzle and pop add in the cauliflower florets. Fry for about 3-4 minutes; you want to get brown spots appearing on the cauliflower.

Pour the suspension of spices over the cauliflower, stir well, then turn the heat right down and put on the lid. Leave to steam for 8 minutes. Put in the diced tomatoes, stir and cook for another 10-15 minutes until the cauliflower is tender.

Lemony leeks and mushrooms
179 calories per serving

One of my favourite suppers. Tasty, filling and easy.

Serves 1 Prep time: 5m Cook time: 12m

1 tbsp olive oil
3 medium leeks, cut into 1cm rings
150g chestnut mushrooms, washed and sliced
juice ½ lemon
freshly ground salt and pepper
sprinkling (10g) parmesan cheese

Heat the oil in a wide lidded frying pan or non-stick saucepan. Add in the leeks and fry on a medium heat for 5 minutes, stirring occasionally until the leeks have some brown bits. Add the mushrooms and continue to fry for a further 2 minutes.

Then add 2 tablespoons water, turn up the heat and put the lid on the pan. Cook for 5 minutes, then remove the lid. If there is any liquid remaining cook with the lid off until the water has boiled off. Remove from the heat and stir in the lemon juice. Serve in a wide bowl topped with salt, pepper and parmesan cheese.

Vegetable curry
181 calories per serving

You could use a pre-mixed madras curry powder instead of the spices.

This could also be made in bigger portions and frozen.

Serves 1 Prep time: 5m Cook time: 40m

1 tsp sunflower oil
½ tsp cumin seeds
½ tsp mustard seeds
½ onion
1 clove garlic
¼ tsp ground coriander
¼ tsp ground cumin
¼ tsp turmeric
½ tsp mild chilli powder
½ tsp salt
½ tin chopped tomatoes
2 handfuls of pre-chopped frozen veg (choose from carrot, peas, green beans, cauliflower, or anything you like!)

Finely chop the onion and garlic. In a deep wide frying pan heat the oil and whole spices (cumin and mustard seeds) together until the spices are just starting to pop. Add the chopped onion and garlic, stir and reduce the heat. Sweat the onions in the pan for up to 10 minutes until they are translucent. Add the ground spices and salt, then stir in thoroughly before adding the chopped tomatoes. Add your choice of veg and then simmer gently for ½ an hour.

Portobello mushrooms with spinach and tomato
195 calories per serving

The quinoa in this recipe adds good quality and filling protein. Who would believe this only has 195 calories?

Serves 1 Prep time: 5m Cook time: 15m

2 Portobello mushrooms
50g fresh spinach (or 2 cubes frozen spinach)
50g ready to eat quinoa or 20g dried quinoa cooked according to packet
2 tsp light crème fraiche
black pepper
1 tomato
½ clove garlic
1 tsp olive oil
10g grated parmesan

Remove the stalks from the mushrooms and set aside. Place the mushrooms on a baking tray and bake for 8 minutes in a pre-heated oven at 200C (180C fan, 400F).

Finely chop the mushroom stalks and dice the tomato. In a frying pan, gently heat the oil and fry the mushroom stalks, garlic and tomato for 3-5 minutes. Then add the spinach, stir and warm through for 2 minutes. Remove from the heat. Stir in the quinoa and crème fraiche. Pile the mixture onto the mushrooms and sprinkle with a little parmesan.

Place the mushrooms back in the oven and cook for a further 6-7 minutes, until the top is golden brown.

Under 300 calories

Sweet potato chilli
212 calories per serving

✓ .good.

Serves 4 Prep time: 5m Cook time: 1h 10m

1 tbsp vegetable oil *4tbsp*
1 large onion, chopped *3 onions*
3 cloves garlic *9 garlic cloves.*
2 fresh green or red chillis *— 1 chilli 3 chillis*
2 large or 3 small sweet potatoes (500g), peeled and cut into big cubes *9 sw-pot*
1 tsp mild chilli powder *3tsp chilli powder*
1 tsp ground cumin *3tsp cumin*
2 tsp paprika *3tsp paprika*
1 tsp cocoa powder *3tsp cocoa* *in bag*
1 tsp salt *3tsp salt*
juice of 1 lime *3 limes*
1 tin tomatoes *3 tin tomatoes*
1 tin red kidney beans *3 tins red kidney beans*

In a large casserole or saucepan gently fry the onions for about 5 minutes.
Chop and de-seed the chillis (to cut it into rounds: cut the top off, hollow out
the seeds with an apple corer or the top of a veg peeler, then cut into
circles.)   Add the chillis and roughly chopped garlic to the onions and fry
for a further couple of minutes.

cook
Add the sweet potato, stir in. Then add the chilli powder, cumin, paprika,
salt and cocoa and stir in. Finally add the tinned tomatoes, kidney beans
(including the water from the can) and lime juice. Stir well. Cook on the
lowest heat for about an hour, lid on.

If you can, leave to cool completely before re-heating to serve – this really
enriches the flavour.

+ 750g rice

Stuffed butternut squash
237 calories per serving

A tasty and filling low-calorie supper. Good for cold Autumn nights.

Serves 2 Prep time: 5m Cook time: 1 hour

3 tsp olive oil
1 butternut squash
1 white onion, chopped into fine half rings
½ red onion, chopped into fine half rings
1 inch thumb ginger
½ tsp cinnamon
½ tsp cumin seeds, crushed in a pestle and mortar
½ tsp paprika
1 tsp salt
2 tbsp sultanas

Halve and de-seed the squash. Score deeply into the squash about 1cm apart from two directions, making checks or diamonds. Add 1 teaspoon of olive oil to each half and roast in the oven at 190C (170C fan, 375F) for 45 minutes.

Gently fry both the red and white onion in the third teaspoon of oil for about 10 minutes. Remove from the heat. Chop the ginger into fine matchsticks and add to the onions. Add spices, salt and sultanas to the onion mixture. Stuff the onions into the roasted squashes and cook for a further 15 minutes.

One pot Thai curry
242 calories per serving

This is called a one pot curry because the rice is cooked within the recipe.
I love to make this for dinner or lunch as it is so flavoursome and satisfying.
As this makes six portions, there's plenty of opportunity to make a big pan
and keep some (it freezes well) for another day.

Serves 6 Prep time: 10m Cook time: 40m

2 chillis, de-seeded and cut into fine rings
6 spring onions, shredded
1 inch thumb ginger, peeled and cut into matchsticks
pinch of mace
1 tsp salt
100g puy lentils
200g wholegrain brown rice
1½ litres chicken or veg stock, fresh preferably or made with 3 stock
cubes
2 tbsp Thai green curry paste
1 can water chestnuts (225g), drained and sliced
1 can reduced fat coconut milk
juice of 2 limes
200g beansprouts
200g young leaf spinach

In a large saucepan place your chillis, spring onions, ginger, mace, salt,
puy lentils and rice. Pour in your stock and bring to the boil. Stir in the
green curry paste. Cook at a low simmer for 30 minutes, or until the lentils
and rice is cooked through.

Now stir in the coconut milk and water chestnuts and simmer for another 5
minutes. Finally add in the beansprouts and spinach, cook for 1-2 minutes,
allowing the spinach to wilt and then serve.

One pot vegetable tagine
247 calories per serving

Like the Thai curry this is an all in one dish that really packs a punch.

Serves 6 Prep time: 10m Cook time: 30m

1 onion, sliced
1 carrot, chopped
1 litre chicken or veg stock, fresh or made with 2 stock cubes
1 tin tomatoes, chopped
2 tsp mild chilli powder
½ tsp cumin
1 tsp salt
200g wild red rice
8 dried apricots, chopped
½ cauliflower, chopped into small florets
1 can chickpeas, drained
200g spinach

In a large casserole dish or saucepan place your onions and carrots. Pour over your stock and bring to the boil. Pour in the red rice and simmer vigorously for 10 minutes.

Next add the tinned tomatoes, spices and salt and stir. Then add dried apricots, cauliflower and chickpeas. Bring back to a simmer and cook for a further 20 minutes. Check that your rice and cauliflower are both cooked through.

Add in the spinach and cook for 1 minute before serving.

J+ Rosie liked
red rice a bit, add more.

Quinoa with red peppers
250 calories per serving

Serves 1 Prep time: 2m Cook time: 20m

1 red pepper, de-seeded and cut into long strips
40g dried quinoa
1 tsp olive oil
½ onion, finely diced
1 garlic clove, finely sliced
1 bay leaf
½ tsp dried oregano
a little chopped fresh parsley if you have it

Put the pepper strips on a grill tray and grill on a medium heat for about 5 minutes each side until tender and black at the edges. In a shallow pan heat the oil gently and fry the onions and garlic for 10 minutes. Rinse the quinoa before stirring into the pan. Add the bay leaf and oregano. Add 200ml water and simmer gently until the water is absorbed – about 8 minutes. Stir the peppers and parsley into the quinoa. Season with salt and pepper.

Broccoli with anchovy dip
251 calories per serving

Works with all kinds of broccoli, including purple sprouting and tender-stem.

Serves 1 Prep time: 2m Cook time: 10m

150g broccoli, cut into florets or stems
1 tbsp olive oil
2 cloves garlic, very finely chopped or crushed
3 anchovy fillets, rinsed and dried

In a small saucepan heat a tiny bit of oil and gently fry the garlic for 2 minutes. Then add the anchovy fillets and mash them slightly with the wooden spoon. Pour in the rest of the oil and cook very, very gently for another 6 minutes.

Meanwhile steam the broccoli for 6 minutes. Serve the dip warm in a small bowl surrounded by the broccoli.

Chicken

Under 200 calories

Herby chicken
185 calories per serving

This makes an extremely tasty and fresh dish. You could substitute the fresh herbs for ½ tsp of mixed dry herbs. Serve with a green vegetable such as broccoli or spinach.

Serves 1 Prep time: 5m Marinate time: 1h Cook time: 25m

1 chicken breast
½ lemon
½ clove garlic (crushed)
Salt and pepper to taste
Mixed fresh herbs e.g. Rosemary, parsley or sage

Use a small oven proof and non-metallic dish that can hold the chicken breast with a little bit of space around it but not much more. Into your dish zest the lemon (wash in hot water and hand soap first if it is waxed) and then add the juice of half the lemon. Add your garlic and salt and pepper and then some roughly chopped herbs.

Snip or score the top of your chicken breast before adding it to the dish. Toss the chicken in the juices and herbs making sure they are covered. Leave them top side up and rub the herbs into the cuts in the chicken as much as you can. Cover with foil and leave to rest for about an hour (½ hour to 3 hours).

Cook in a pre-heated oven for 20 minutes at 180C (170C fan or 360F) covered and then uncover and cook at 220C (210C fan or 430F) for another 5 minutes.

Sticky Thai chicken
205 calories per serving

Serves 1 Prep time: 5m Marinate time: 1h Cook time: 10m

1 chicken breast skinned and chopped into big chunks
1 cloves garlic
1 small thumb ginger
1 tbsp soy sauce
½ tsp honey

Prepare the marinade by grating the garlic and ginger on the fine side of the grater. Mix in the soy sauce and honey. Add the chicken to the marinade and leave for at least one hour. Remove the chicken from the marinade and grill (on a medium heat) for 5-6 minutes each side.

Under 300 calories

Creamy chicken curry
245 calories per serving

Packed with flavour this recipe serves 4 but can be frozen in batches.

Serves 4 Prep time: 10m Cook time: 55m

1 tbsp vegetable oil
1 tsp cumin seeds
¼ tsp black mustard seeds (if available)
2 onions, finely sliced
3 chicken breasts, cut into chunks
2 tsp turmeric
¼ tsp ground cinnamon
½ tsp ground ginger
½ tsp mild chilli powder
1 tsp salt
1 can tomatoes
125ml water
100g baby spinach
2 tbsp mango chutney
4 tbsp (60ml) light crème fraiche

Heat the oil on a medium heat in a casserole or lidded saucepan. Add the cumin and mustard seeds and fry for 1 minute or until they start to sizzle. Turn the heat down and add the onion, fry gently for 5 minutes. Add in the rest of the spices and the salt, stir thoroughly. Add in the chicken, stir and then immediately add the tin of tomatoes and the water. Bring to the boil and simmer for 40 minutes.

Stir the spinach into the curry and cook for 1-2 minutes, allowing it to wilt. Stir in the mango chutney and crème fraiche. Warm through.

Chicken in tomato sauce
255 calories per serving

The tomato sauce is very versatile and can also be used on pasta and pizza. This recipe serves four but if you make the sauce for four you can keep or freeze some and use ¼ of the sauce with one chicken breast.

Serves 4 Prep time: 5m Cook time: 1h 10m

2 cloves garlic, finely sliced
1 tsp olive oil
2 tins tomatoes, whole not chopped
2 red peppers, de-seeded and chopped
1 courgette, skinned and chopped
4 chicken breasts, skinless | = | 75 c

In a wide saucepan gently heat the oil and toss in the garlic. Lightly fry for 2-3 minutes. As they are just starting to turn brown add the tins of tomatoes, peppers and courgette. Bring to simmering point and then turn heat down a little, making sure it continues to bubble. Simmer like this for ½ hour, stirring occasionally. Then break up the tomatoes with a wooden spoon and continue to cook for a further ¼ hour.

To make a smooth sauce transfer to a liquidiser and whizz for approx 1 minute. (You can of course skip this step and choose a more textured sauce.) In the same saucepan (or a smaller pan if you are just cooking one piece) place the whole pieces of chicken flat on the bottom of the pan. Pour over the sauce so it covers the chicken generously. Bring the sauce up to a simmer and cook for 25 minutes on a gentle heat until the chicken is cooked. If the pan looks dry or the chicken becomes uncovered you should add a little water and stir in.

Chicken with brown mushrooms
284 calories per serving

A lovely autumnal and earthy dish. Ideal served with ¼ savoy cabbage (27 calories).

Serves 1 Prep time: 5m Soak time: 30m Cook time: 15m

1 tsp olive oil   *1t = 41 cal*
½ leek, chopped into rings   *½ leek = 11 cal*
1 chicken breast cut into about 6 pieces   *170 gr = 175 Cal*
½ clove garlic
About 6 brown mushrooms sliced *} ord mush = 11 Cal*
2 dried porcini mushrooms
1 tbsp Cooking sherry
1 tbsp light crème fraiche   *ord mary creme frache = 1T = 45 C*

Put the porcini mushrooms in a mug with ⅓ cup boiling water. Leave to soak for ½ hour. In a large frying pan heat the oil and fry the leeks and chicken on a medium heat for 8 minutes. Stir a few times but not too often.

Turn to a low heat and add the crushed garlic and brown mushrooms. Fry for 4 minutes.

Turn to a medium heat. Add the cooking sherry (it should sizzle a bit). Add the porcini mushrooms and the liquid you soaked them in, discarding the grit at the bottom of the cup. Add salt and pepper to taste. Simmer gently for 2 minutes before finally adding the crème fraiche and serving.

Chicken with orange and black olives
284 calories per serving

Delicious served with a serving of spinach (14 calories for a 50g portion).

Serves 1 Prep time: 5m Cook time: 15m

1 skinless chicken breast
50ml chicken stock (fresh, or made with half a stock cube)
½ small orange
Approx 6 pitted black olives
Pinch of dried sage
1 tsp olive oil

In a lidded frying pan gently heat the olive oil for a few minutes before adding the chicken breast. Cook for 2 minutes on each side on a medium to high heat. Turn the heat down and add the stock, the orange (quarter it, cut out the pith, cut the flesh out of the skin and roughly slice), olives and sage.

Put the lid on and cook for 10 minutes. Remove the lid and raise the temperature for 2 minutes to reduce the sauce a little.

Hot chicken curry
288 calories per serving

Serves 1 Prep time: 10m Marinate time: 30m Cook time: 1h

½ onion
1 clove garlic
1 chilli
1 thumb ginger
1 skinless chicken breast
1 tbsp low fat yoghurt
¼ tsp ground cumin
¼ tsp ground coriander
¼ tsp turmeric
½ tsp salt
¼ tsp garam masala
½ tin tomatoes
a few sprays of light sunflower oil spray such as Fry Light

Peel the onion, garlic and ginger, and de-seed the chilli. Put all of them into a food processor and whizz until finely chopped. Place half the onion mix in a bowl and mix in the yoghurt. Cube the chicken and add to the yoghurt mixture. Leave for ½ hour.

Meanwhile in an oven proof pan heat 3 or 4 sprays of sunflower oil spray and add the rest of the onion mixture. Fry gently for 3 minutes, stirring now and again. Add all the spices and salt. In the processor (no need to clean after onions) whizz the tomatoes. Add the tomatoes to the pan and cook on lowest heat uncovered for ½ hour.

Add the chicken and yoghurt to the pan stir and cover. Cook in preheated oven at 190C (170C fan, 370F) for 30 minutes.

Moroccan chicken casserole
291 calories per serving

An unusual and interesting mix of flavours. Ideal served with spinach (15 calories in a 50g serving).

Serves 1 Prep time: 10m Marinate time: 2h Cook time: 15m

1 clove garlic
Pinch of rock salt
½ tsp paprika
¼ tsp turmeric
¼ tsp cumin seed
1 chicken breast
1 tsp olive oil
½ onion
½ lemon
Pinch saffron (optional)
5 green pitted olives

First you need to make a rub for the chicken. In a pestle and mortar mash up the garlic with a pinch of rock salt and the cumin seeds. Then add the paprika and turmeric.

Score the chicken and then rub the mix all over the chicken. Leave for a few hours. 2 hours minimum, 4 ideal or all day.

In a smallish lidded frying pan or saucepan fry the finely sliced onions slowly in the oil for about 5 minutes uncovered. Remove the wax from the lemon by washing in hot water with soap. Cut four very thin slices of lemon. Layer the lemon on top of the onion and put the chicken breasts on top of that. Add enough water to just cover the chicken and bring to boil. Reduce to a low simmer and cook for 15 minutes with the lid on the pan.

not too much water.

Jerusalem artichokes, leeks and chicken
294 calories per serving

Jerusalem artichokes are incredibly tasty and good for you. If you can get hold of them (normally best in October and November) this is my favourite recipe for them. Note that as the artichokes are quite substantial, I have reduced the amount of chicken.

Serves 2 Prep time: 10m Cook time: 15m

1 tbsp olive oil
6-8 Jerusalem artichokes (300g)
1 chicken breast, cut into small strips
1 large or 2 small leeks, cut into small rings.
juice of 1 lemon

First prepare your artichokes by cutting off the knobbly bits and then peeling. Cut into fine slices (not more than 2mm thick). Heat the oil on a high heat in a large lidded frying pan. Toss in the artichokes and fry for 2 minutes.

Next add the leeks, turn the heat down, add 4 tablespoons water and place the lid on the pan. Cook for 6 minutes.

After this remove the lid from the pan and stir.

Turn the heat back up to medium high and when hot add the chicken pieces. Cook for another 5-6 minutes, stirring occasionally, until the chicken is cooked and all ingredients are browning nicely. Remove from the heat and stir in the lemon juice.

Fish

Under 200 calories

Prawn cocktail
160 calories per serving

Serves 1 Prep time: 5m

100g jumbo king prawns, cooked
1 little gem lettuce, quartered
2 inches cucumber, cut into chunky sticks
4 tsp extra light mayonnaise
1 tsp reduced sugar and salt ketchup
dash of Worcestershire sauce
1 tsp lemon juice
a little paprika

Mix together the mayonnaise, ketchup, Worcestershire sauce and lemon juice. Arrange the prawns on a plate with the gem lettuce and cucumber. Put the cocktail sauce separately as a dip. Sprinkle the dip with a little paprika.

Lemon sole with a herb crust
185 calories per serving

Serves 2 Prep time: 5m Cook time: 12m

2 lemon sole fillets (approximately 130g each)
1 thin slice / ½ thick slice granary bread, crusts removed
1 lemon
2 tsp fresh herbs, shredded (oregano, parsley, basil or a mixture of all three)

Make breadcrumbs from the bread. Either blend in a food processor or chop into very small chunks with a bread-knife. Remove the wax from the lemon by washing in warm soapy water and dry. Finely grate the zest of the lemon into the breadcrumbs. Add in the fresh herbs and a little freshly ground salt and pepper. Stir in the juice of ½ lemon.

Put the fish fillets on a baking tray and gently press the bread-crumb mixture over the top. Cook in a pre-heated oven at 220C (200C fan, 430F) for 10-12 minutes. Serve on a bed of salad leaves with a lemon wedge on the side.

Fresh pesto cod
187 calories per serving

Serve with fresh spinach, lightly cooked and drizzled with lemon juice and black pepper.

Serves 1 Prep time: 10m Cook time: 15m

1 cod fillet, skinless
20g fresh basil leaves
pinch of sea salt
1 tsp pine nuts
5g parmesan

Roughly chop your fresh basil. Place in a pestle and mortar with the sea salt and grind until you have a mushy paste. Add the pine nuts and pound again. Add a little water (2 teaspoons) and pound/stir once more. Spread the paste over your cod and place in an oven-proof dish. Grate a little (5g) parmesan over the top. Cook in a pre-heated oven at 220C (200C fan, 430F) for 15 minutes.

Fish fingers and salad
195 calories per serving

I know, I know, this is NOT a recipe. But the kids and I eat this quite happily at least once a fortnight. They just add ketchup. If you haven't eaten fish fingers in a while...try them, it should take you right back to childhood!

2 fish fingers
Standard salad (see page 47) including dressing

Under 300 calories

Coconut and cumin prawns
206 calories per serving

This dish is also excellent made with crayfish if you can get hold of any.
Serve with a salad of tomato, red onion, coriander and lemon juice.

Serves 2 Prep time: 5m Cook time: 15m

1 tsp sunflower oil
½ tsp cumin seeds
½ onion, finely diced
2 tomatoes, diced
½ tsp salt
1 green chilli, de-seeded and sliced
¼ tsp ground turmeric
¼ tsp mild chilli powder
100ml (¼ can) light coconut milk
200g raw prawns, shelled (defrosted if frozen)

Heat the oil on a medium heat in a wide, lidded frying pan. When it's hot toss in the cumin seeds and when they are sizzling add in the onion and stir. Fry gently until golden – about 5 minutes.

Turn the heat to low. Add the tomatoes, salt, chilli, ground turmeric and chilli powder. Stir well. Gently cook for 5 minutes. Stir in the coconut milk, heat for another 3 minutes. Stir in the prawns, and finally cook with the lid on for another 3 minutes.

Cajun salmon
213 calories per serving

A simple way to jazz up a piece of salmon. Serve with a salad.

Serves 1 Prep time: 1m Cook time: 15m

1 skinless salmon fillet
1 tsp shop-bought Cajun seasoning

Pre-heat oven to 220C (200C fan, 430F). Place 2 salmon fillets on a baking tray. Rub a teaspoon of cajun spices over each fillet. Cook for 15 minutes.

Chunky cod with tomatoes and spinach
248 calories per serving

Serves 2 Prep time: 10m Cook time: 20m

2 cod fillets, skinless (about 125g each)
sea salt crystals
2 tsp olive oil
2 tbsp capers
3 tomatoes, diced
½ onion
1 clove garlic, finely chopped
pinch chilli flakes
100g baby spinach

Cut each piece of cod into 3 pieces. Rub a little of the sea salt onto each of the cod chunks. Heat 1 tsp oil in a small frying pan and add the capers. Fry for 4-5 minutes until they turn crispy but not burnt. Heat the remaining teaspoon of oil in a heavy casserole dish. Add the onion and garlic and cook over a low heat for 10 minutes until translucent.

Add the chilli flakes and tomato, stir, and lay the cod pieces on top with a scattering of freshly ground pepper.

Place the lid on the casserole dish and steam the fish for 10 minutes.

When the fish is cooked, remove the fish from the pan and set aside. Put the spinach into the casserole dish, stir and put the lid on. Leave to wilt for 1-2 minutes. Then stir again, transfer to plates and put the cod on the top. Scatter over the crispy capers.

Salmon and cod fishcakes
256 calories per serving

Serves 4 Prep time: 10m Cook time: 40m

2 skinless salmon fillets
1 skinless cod fillet
1 bay leaf
a little dill
200ml white wine
100g light mayonnaise
100g breadcrumbs

Place the fish in a baking dish with the bay leaf and dill. Pour over the white wine and cover with foil. Cook in a pre-heated oven at 190C (170C fan, 370F) for 22 minutes. Allow to cool and drain and dry on some kitchen paper.

Using a fork, break up the fish into smaller pieces. Then add in the breadcrumbs, mayonnaise and some salt and pepper. Combine thoroughly. Shape the fish mixture into balls, making 12-14 in total. Place the balls on a non-stick baking tray and flatten into cakes with the palm of your hand.

Cook in a pre-heated oven at 220C (200C fan or 430F) for 12-15 minutes until starting to brown.

Scallops with garlic tomatoes
258 calories per serving

Serves 1 Prep time: 5m Cook time: 10m

80g fresh green beans
6 cherry tomatoes, halved
1 tsp olive oil
1 clove garlic, very finely sliced
100g scallops

Cook the green beans by boiling in water for 4 minutes. In a frying pan gently heat the oil. Toss in the garlic and after 1 minute add the cherry tomatoes. Fry gently for 4 minutes. Remove tomato mixture from the pan and turn the heat up to medium high. Cook the scallops for 30 seconds to 1 minute each side until opaque and just cooked through.

Put the green beans on a warm plate and arrange the scallops over the top. Scatter with black pepper. Finally place the tomatoes and garlic on the top.

Oven baked tandoori salmon
281 calories per serving

Serve with broccoli or peas.

Serves 1 Prep time: 5m Marinate time: 1h Cook time: 15m

1 skinless salmon fillet
50g low fat natural yoghurt
Juice of half lemon
1 small thumb ginger
1 clove garlic
½ tsp ground cumin
½ tsp chilli powder
¼ tsp turmeric
¼ tsp garam masala
½ tsp salt

Grate the ginger and garlic on the fine side of the grater. Mix all the ingredients except the salmon together. Put the salmon in a plastic bag and mix in the yoghurt paste. Marinate for an hour. Cook in a pre-heated oven at 220C (200C fan, 430F) for 15 minutes.

Spicy Indian prawns and rice
290 calories per serving

Serves 2 Pre-time: 5m Cook time: 25m

80g basmati rice
2 tsp sunflower oil
¼ tsp cumin seeds
½ cinnamon stick
2 cloves
1 bay leaf
½ onion, finely chopped
1 birds eye chilli, de-seeded and sliced
4 cloves garlic, finely chopped
½ tsp mild chilli powder
1 tsp paprika
½ tsp salt
2 fresh tomatoes, diced
150g cooked prawns

Cook the rice by your preferred method and leave to cool.

Heat the oil in a wide frying pan on a medium high heat. Add the cumin seeds, bay leaf, cinnamon and cloves. Fry for 1 minute before adding the chopped onion, chillies and garlic. Fry gently for 5 minutes until the onions are starting to brown.

Add the tomatoes, chilli powder, paprika and salt. Continue cooking on a low heat for a further 7 minutes. Add the prawns and rice and cook gently for 5 more minutes until they are warmed through.

Haddock with olives and tomatoes
293 calories per serving

Serve with green beans or spinach.

Serves 1 Prep time: 2m Cook time: 12m

1 large haddock fillet, skinless and boneless
1 tbsp black olive paste or meze
1 tsp extra virgin olive oil
4 cherry tomatoes, quartered
2 basil leaves, shredded
juice of ½ lime

Spread the olive puree on both sides of the fish. Heat a non-stick frying pan on a medium high heat and place the haddock in the pan. Cook for 10-15 minutes, turning once. The cooking time depends on the thickness of the fillet. Remove the fish to a warm plate. Add the tomatoes, olive oil, basil and lime juice to the pan. Heat for 2 minutes and serve poured over the haddock.

Steamed salmon with Chinese vegetables
296 calories per serving

Serves 1 Prep time: 10m Cook time: 10m

¼ onion, thinly sliced
1 salmon fillet, skinless and boneless
¼ savoy cabbage, sliced
½ small carrot (cut into small strips)
½ fennel bulb (cut into small strips)
1 small thumb ginger, grated
1 tbsp Soy sauce
2 drops nam pla (Fish sauce)
2 drops Sesame oil

In a large lidded frying pan add about ½ cm depth of water and bring to the boil. Add the onion, carrot and fennel and put the lid on. Continue on full heat for 5 minutes. Check water levels and add the cabbage. Put the lid back on and cook for a further 5 minutes on a medium high flame.

Add the grated ginger, soy and fish sauce and stir in. If necessary add a little more water too. Cut the salmon into big chunks and place on top of the veg. Add the 2 drops of sesame oil. Put the lid back on and steam for 6 minutes. Serve carefully to stop the salmon breaking up.

[handwritten:] Haddock
100 gr = 74
120 = ±90

Haddock with Sauce Vierge
300 calories per serving

Serves 2 Prep time: 15m Cook time: 20m

2 haddock fillets, skinless and boneless (approximately 130g each)
2 tbsp extra virgin olive oil   *[handwritten:]* 30 ml = 200 cal .
½ tsp ground cumin
½ tsp ground coriander
3 sprigs saffron
1 red pepper, de-seeded and finely chopped   *[handwritten:]* 100 gr = 30 cal
1 tomato, finely chopped   *[handwritten:]* 80gr x 2   160 gr = ±30 cal
1 tsp fresh mint, finely shredded
1 tsp fresh coriander, finely shredded

Place the saffron in a small cup or bowl and pour over a small amount of boiling water. Leave to steep for 10 minutes.

Heat a small frying pan to a medium high heat. Put the red peppers in the frying pan with no oil. Chargrill the red peppers for about 4 minutes each side. They should be tender and a little black on the outside.

Put the haddock fillets on a baking tray and sprinkle with salt and pepper. Bake in a pre-heated oven at 200C (180C fan, 390F) for 15-18 minutes until cooked through.

In a small saucepan combine the olive oil, spices, saffron (including the soaking liquid), cooked red pepper, tomato and fresh herbs. Heat for two minutes very gently until the sauce reaches blood temperature. Serve poured over the baked fish.

Teriyaki salmon
310 calories per serving

Flavoursome one-dish meal.

Serves 1 Prep time: 5m Marinate time: 2h Cook time: 15m

1 skinless salmon fillet
1 inch thumb ginger, grated
1 clove garlic, grated or crushed
1 tsp nam pla or fish sauce
1 tsp soy sauce
½ tsp sesame oil
1 tsp honey
120ml water
1 Pak choi, chopped
6 mushrooms, sliced
¼ savoy cabbage, finely sliced

First make your marinade by mixing together the ginger, garlic, nam pla, soy sauce, sesame oil, honey, water. Put the marinade in a wide bowl. Put the salmon in the bowl and scoop up some of the marinade to cover all the salmon. Leave for about 2 hours.

To cook your salmon place on a medium high grill for about 5 minutes each side until golden brown and cooked through. Leave the left over marinade aside for cooking the vegetables.

To prepare the pak choi, mushrooms and cabbage, take a wide lidded saucepan and tip in the marinade. Put the lid on. On a medium high flame, heat the marinade for several minutes until bubbling fast. Add in your chopped veg and stir. Quickly replace the lid and steam for 5 minutes.

Meat

Under 200 calories

Kale with bacon and tomato
197 calories per serving

Easy to rustle up, this is warming and filling.

Serves 1 Prep time: 5m Cook time: 20m

2 sprays of light cooking oil
½ onion, diced
2 low fat bacon rashers, cut into strips
¼ can haricot beans
1 tomato, diced
80g (or as much as you can fit in the pan) curly leaf kale

In a wide lidded saucepan fry the onion slowly in the spray oil for 5 minutes. Then turn the heat up to medium and add the bacon. Fry for a further 5 minutes, turning now and again. Now add the haricot beans, tomato and 3 tablespoons water. Stir and then add the kale on the top. Put the lid on the pan, turn the heat up high and cook for 6-8 minutes until the kale is cooked and tender.

Autumn lamb stew
198 calories per serving

The following recipe serves eight people. It is therefore suitable for cooking in bulk and freezing in individual portions.

Serves 8 Prep time: 15m Cook time: 2h 30m

600g lean diced lamb
2 tbsp olive oil
1 onion
2 carrots
4 celery stalks
2 cloves garlic
200ml red wine
1 small swede
2 tbsp tom purée
2 can tomatoes
2 bay leaves
500ml veg or chicken stock

Heat the oil in a large oven proof casserole. Add the lamb and roughly chopped onions. Stir. Cook for 5 minutes until you get a couple of burnt bits. Roughly chop all veg (this is a big chunk casserole). Add the sliced garlic and chopped veg. Stir and cook for another 5 minutes.

Add the rest of the ingredients and bring to the boil. Simmer gently for 30 minutes. Either transfer to a slow cooker for about 8 hours or else cook with the lid on for about 4 hours at 140C (120C fan, 275F) or 2 hours at a very low simmer.

Kofta lamb meatballs
200 calories per serving

You could also make this with beef mince. Serve on a bed of crispy salad leaves with a wedge of lemon.

Serves 4 Prep time: 10m Cook time: 20m

400g extra lean lamb mince
1 onion, peeled and chopped
2 tsp ground cumin
2 garlic cloves, peeled
pinch cayenne pepper
handful of fresh coriander leaves
1 tsp baking powder
1 tsp salt
1 tbsp olive oil

Place all the ingredients except the olive oil in a food processor and blend. The mixture needs to be sticking together but not smooth.

Take a small handful of the mixture and make into a small oval ball (the kofta). The mixture should make about 16 koftas. Brush each kofta with a little olive oil and place on a non-stick baking tray. Pre-heat the oven to 190C (170C fan, 370F) and cook for 20 minutes until turning brown and crispy.

Under 300 calories

Sweet and sour pork
218 calories per serving

Serve with a green vegetable such as broccoli, green beans or spinach.

Serves 1 Prep time: 2m Cook time: 15m

1 lean, trimmed pork steak (approx 125g)
salt and pepper
½ tsp brown sugar
½ tsp English mustard
1 tsp red wine vinegar
½ tsp ketchup
2 tbsp water

Season the pork with salt and pepper. Heat a frying pan to a medium heat and add the pork steak. You want it to be just sizzling the whole time. Cook for approximately 7 minutes each side.

Meanwhile make the dressing by simply mixing the rest of the ingredients together in a small bowl. Add a generous quantity of salt and pepper to the sauce as well.

When you are happy that the pork is well cooked turn the heat right down and pour in the sauce over the pork. It should sizzle frantically at first and then calm down to a gentle bubble. Cook for a further minute or two.

Quick fried beef with Salsa Verde
224 calories per serving

Beef escalopes are not expensive, are easy to cook and have only 160 calories each. Try serving with green beans.

Serves 2 Prep time: 10m Infuse time: 15m+ Cook time: 5m

2 leaves flat leaf parsley
2 basil leaves
2 mint leaves
1 large/ 2 small gherkins
1 garlic clove, peeled
1 tsp capers
2 anchovy fillets
1 tsp red wine vinegar
juice of ½ lime
1 tsp Dijon mustard
1 tsp extra virgin olive oil
2 lean beef escalopes (up to 150g each)

Coarsely chop the herbs, gherkins, garlic and anchovy fillets. Place in a bowl with the capers. Add in the red wine vinegar, lime juice, mustard and olive oil. Add in a tablespoon water and some ground black pepper. Stir and set aside (the flavours develop best if left for up to an hour).

Heat a heavy based frying pan to a medium high heat. Add in your escalopes and fry for 1-2 minutes each side, depending on how you like your beef.

Lamb tagine
227 calories per serving

This tagine is packed with flavour and is a firm favourite in our house.

Serves 8 Prep time: 15m Cook time: 2h 45m

2 tbsp oil
600g extra lean diced lamb
1 large / 2 small onions, sliced
2 garlic cloves, finely sliced
2 sticks celery, diced
1 carrot, diced
4 sun-dried tomatoes, re-hydrated in boiling water if dried
2 tsp mild chilli powder
½ tsp cumin powder
2 tsp salt
1 tin tomatoes
1 tin chickpeas, drained
8 dried apricots (100g), chopped
12 black pitted olives
juice of 1 lime
juice of 1 lemon

Heat the oil in a large lidded casserole dish and fry the lamb in 2 batches. Cook for 2 minutes each side until starting to brown and crisp. Remove the lamb to a plate and set aside.

Reduce the heat in the pan and add the onions and garlic. Cook slowly for 5 minutes.

Add the carrot and celery and continue heating slowly for another 5 minutes. Stir in the spices and salt. Put the meat back in the pan. Then add the tomatoes, chickpeas, apricots and olives. Bring up to simmer and cook with the lid off for ½ hour.

Put the lid on and cook in the oven for 2 hours at 180C (160C fan or 360F) or for 8 hours in a slow cooker. At the end of the cooking time, stir in the lemon and lime juice.

Chilli con carne
235 calories per serving

This chilli tastes even better if chilled or frozen and re-heated.

Serves 8 Prep time: 10m Cook time: 2h 30 minimum

1 tsp sunflower oil
1 large onion (or 2 small) chopped
3 cloves garlic, roughly chopped
2 fresh green or red chillies (2)
800g lean beef mince
1 tsp mild chilli powder — needs two .
1 tsp ground cumin
2 tsp paprika
1 tsp cocoa powder
1 tsp salt
Juice of 1 lime
1 tin tomatoes
1 tin red kidney beans

In a large casserole or saucepan gently fry the onions in the oil for about 5 minutes, until translucent. Chop and de-seed the chillies.

Add the chillies and garlic to the onions and fry for a further couple of minutes. Add the mince and continue frying until browned. Then add the chilli powder, cumin, paprika, salt and cocoa and stir in. Finally add the lime juice, tinned tomatoes and kidney beans. Simmer gently for 30 minutes.

Add a little water if it looks like it might dry out during cooking. Transfer to a slow cooker for about 8 hours or else cook for about 4 hours at 140C (120C fan, 275F) or 2 hours at a very low simmer.

Texan chilli beef stew
238 calories per serving

The following recipe serves eight people. It is therefore suitable for cooking in bulk and freezing in individual portions.

Serves 8 Prep time: 10m Cook time: 2h 30 minimum

2 tbsp sunflower oil
800g diced casserole beef
1 tsp flaked chilli
1 tsp ground cumin
2 tsp paprika
1 tsp salt
3 cloves garlic – finely chopped
1 can tomatoes
1 butternut squash
1 sweet potato

large blue Le Creucet

Toss the chopped beef in the spices and seasoning until it is well covered.

Heat the oil in a large oven-proof saucepan and wait until it is really hot.

Add the beef to the saucepan and brown all over. You may have to do this in 2 batches. It is likely to stick to the bottom but don't worry!

Add the chopped garlic and fry for another minute. Add the tinned tomatoes and the veg and bring to simmering point. Simmer gently for 30 minutes. Add a little water if it looks like it might dry out during cooking.

Transfer to a slow cooker for about 8 hours or else cook with the lid on for about 4 hours at 140C (120C fan, 275F) or 2 hours at a very low simmer.

+ 140 cal Chickpeas
   + this treates.

+ 160   punes 100g   → 280 per serving.

Beef in mushrooms and wine
294 calories per serving

Serve with any green vegetable.

Serves 2 Prep time: 5m Cook time: 25m

4 dried porcini mushrooms
1 tsp vegetable oil
1 onion, finely diced
1 garlic clove, finely chopped
8 chestnut or button mushrooms, washed and sliced
200ml red wine
1 tsp cornflour
2 lean beef escalopes (up to 150g each)

Put the porcini mushrooms in ¼ cup of boiling water and leave to soak for at least 15 minutes. In a frying pan heat the oil gently and add the onions. Cook gently for 10 minutes. Add the sliced mushrooms and garlic and fry gently for a further 5 minutes. Remove the mushroom mixture from the pan and set aside.

Turn up the heat to medium high and sear the beef for about 1 minute each side. Reduce the heat and reintroduce the mushroom mix. Stir in the red wine. Finely slice the porcini mushrooms and add them, together with their soaking liquid. Bring the mixture to a gentle simmer. Mix the cornflour with a little water and add to the pan. Stir well. Simmer for 5-10 minutes.

Paprika pork casserole
307 calories per serving

This recipe makes eight portions. It is suitable for freezing.

Serves 8 Prep time: 10m Cook time: 2h 30 minimum

2 tbsp oil
600g diced lean pork
1 large onion
2 peppers (red, yellow or green)
2 cloves garlic, chopped
1 tsp hot paprika
1 tsp smoked paprika
2 tins tomatoes
1 tsp salt
1 chicken stock cube
200ml light crème fraiche

Toss the pork in some salt and pepper. In a casserole dish that can go in the oven fry off the pork in small batches in very hot oil and set aside when starting to turn brown.

Roughly chop the onion and sauté gently in the left over oil for about 5 minutes.

Then add the peppers, garlic and the meat. Stir in the 2 types of paprika and then add the tinned tomatoes, crumbled stock cube and a little salt. Simmer gently for 30 minutes. Add a little water if it looks like it might dry out during cooking.

Transfer to a slow cooker for about 8 hours or else cook with the lid on for about 4 hours at 140C (120C fan, 275F) or 2 hours at a very low simmer. Stir in the crème fraiche before serving.

Sweet treats

Under 150 calories

Chocolate dipped strawberries
90 calories per serving

Makes 4 servings Prep time: 10m Chilling time: 30m

250g strawberries
50g dark 70% chocolate

First remove the stalks from the strawberries, halve any big ones, wash them and dry on some kitchen paper. Prepare a large plate or baking sheet by covering it with greaseproof paper.

Break the chocolate into chunks and put into a small heat proof bowl. Place the bowl over a saucepan of simmering water. Stir occasionally and when the chocolate has completely melted move the pan and bowl together to where you want to dip your strawberries.

Hold the fat end of a strawberry and dip the tip into the melted chocolate. You want the strawberry to be about one third covered. Then place the strawberry, tip up (if possible!) on the greaseproof paper. Repeat with all the strawberries. Place the strawberries in the fridge to set.

Meringue with strawberry compote
100 calories per serving

Meringue nests bought from the supermarket are fat free and have only 52 calories. The strawberry compote lasts for up to 3 days covered in the fridge.

Makes 4 servings of compote

250g strawberries
2 tbsp caster sugar
juice of 1 lemon

1 meringue nest per person

Hull and wash the strawberries. Cut into thin slices (2-4mm). Place the strawberries in a bowl and cover with sugar. Squeeze over the lemon juice and stir in well. Leave for at least ½ hour for the flavours to combine.

Serve chilled piled onto a meringue.

Apricot cereal bars
139 calories per serving

Finding a snack to eat on the go can be a real challenge. These apricot cereal bars are nutritious and sustaining. They also keep for up to 2 weeks in an air-tight container. An individual slice can easily be wrapped in cling film for eating wherever and whenever.

Makes 16 servings Prep time: 10m Cook time: 45m

1 can light condensed milk (397g)
250g rolled porridge oats
100g dried apricots
2-3 sprays sunflower oil spray

Line an 8" square cake tin with greaseproof paper and spray with sunflower oil spray to prevent sticking. In a small pan, warm the condensed milk on a low heat for about 5 minutes. You want it to be warm but not boiling.

Meanwhile, chop the apricots into small pieces and mix into the oats in a large mixing bowl.

When the condensed milk has just started to steam, pour it in over the oats and apricots and mix thoroughly. Scoop this mixture into your cake tin and bake in a pre-heated oven at 160C (140C fan or 320F) for 45 minutes.

When you remove the tin from the oven, immediately transfer the cooked oats to a chopping board and cut into 16 squares with a very sharp knife. Then leave to cool completely on the chopping board.

Calorie counting reference

Although by no means extensive this covers a lot of the food that you are likely to eat on your diet days.

Lower calorie carbs

Basmati rice	40g serving (dry weight)	141 calories
Couscous	40g serving (dry weight)	150 calories
New potatoes	180g, 4 medium new potatoes	135 calories
Pitta bread	1 pitta	161 calories
Oatcake	2 oatcakes	94 calories
Quinoa	40g serving (dry weight)	147 calories

Meat, fish and eggs

Egg	1 large egg	89 cals
Egg white	1 egg white	18 cals
Chicken	1 chicken breast, skin off (approximately 170g)	175 cals
Salmon	1 avg salmon fillet, skin off (approximately 120g)	213 cals
Fish fingers	3 fish fingers	175 cals
Lean minced beef	100g serving	183 cals
Pork chop	1 pork chop (approximately 170g)	437 cals
Lamb chop	1 lamb chop (approximately 100g)	277 cals
Cod	1 cod fillet (130g)	127 cals
Prawns	1 portion (75g)	60 cals

Vegetables and salad

Lettuce	¼ iceberg lettuce	14 cals
Cucumber	100g (2 inches, 5cm)	10 cals
Tomato	2 medium tomatoes	44 cals
Broccoli	100g serving	33 cals
Savoy Cabbage	100g serving, ¼ cabbage	27 cals
Onion	1 med onion, 180g	55 cals
Red pepper	1 med pepper, 100g	32 cals
Green pepper	1 med pepper, 100g	15 cals
Mushrooms	1 normal serving (100g)	13 cals
Leeks	1 normal serving (100g)	23 cals
Pak choi	1 normal serving (100g)	11 cals
Kale	1 normal serving (50g)	16 cals
Spinach	1 normal serving (50g)	14 cals
Peas	1 normal serving (80g)	54 cals
Courgette	1 med courgette (150g)	33 cals
Green beans	1 normal serving (100g)	35 cals

∴ 350 = 246 c

Other

Baked beans	1 can (415g)	328 cals
Tinned tomatoes	1 can (400g)	84 cals

Banana   medium   105
Apple   small 80   med 95
Clementine   32

Sources & bibliography

Healthy fellow interview with Dr Krista Varady

http://www.healthyfellow.com/511/alternate-day-fasting-interview-part-1/

http://www.healthyfellow.com/517/dr-krista-varady-interview-part-2/

The American Journal of Clinical Nutrition "Alternate Day Fasting and Chronic Disease Prevention: A Review of Animal and Human Trials"

http://ajcn.nutrition.org/content/86/1/7.full

The power of intermittent fasting

http://www.bbc.co.uk/news/health-19112549

The American Journal of Clinical Nutrition "Alternate-day fasting: effects on body weight, body composition, energy metabolism"

http://ajcn.nutrition.org/content/81/1/69.full

The 5:2 diet: can it help you lose weight and live longer?

http://www.telegraph.co.uk/lifestyle/9480451/The-52-diet-can-it-help-you-lose-weight-and-live-longer.html

Fasting can help protect against brain diseases, scientists say

http://www.guardian.co.uk/society/2012/feb/18/fasting-protect-brain-diseases-scientists

Bibliography

Fuhrman, Joel, Fasting and Eating for Health, 1995

New Covent Garden Food Co, *A Soup for every day*, 2010

Shelton, Herbert M, *Fasting can save your life*, 1964

Reviews

If this book has inspired you to make a success of the 5:2 diet please leave your story as a review on amazon.co.uk. You may just inspire others to join in too.

Disclaimer

The information provided in this book is designed to provide helpful information on the subjects discussed. This book is not meant to be used, nor should it be used, to diagnose or treat any medical condition. For diagnosis or treatment of any medical problem consult your own doctor.

The publisher and author are not responsible for any specific health or allergy needs that may require medical supervision and are not liable for any damages or negative consequences from any treatment, action, application or preparation, to any person reading or following the information in this book. References are provided for informational purposes only and do not constitute endorsement of any websites or other sources. Readers should be aware that the websites listed in this book may change.

Current medical opinion suggest that the benefits of fasting are unproven. Until they are proven you undertake fasting at your own risk. There are certain medical conditions that would make fasting dangerous and fasting should definitely not be undertaken if you suffer from diabetes or are pregnant or breastfeeding. This list is not authoritative and there may be other medical conditions under which you should not attempt fasting. If in doubt consult your doctor.

Index

Printed in Great Britain
by Amazon.co.uk, Ltd.,
Marston Gate.